PALEO
COOKBOOK

Over 200 Easy and Tasty Recipes
for Complete Wellness

ALEX HENRY

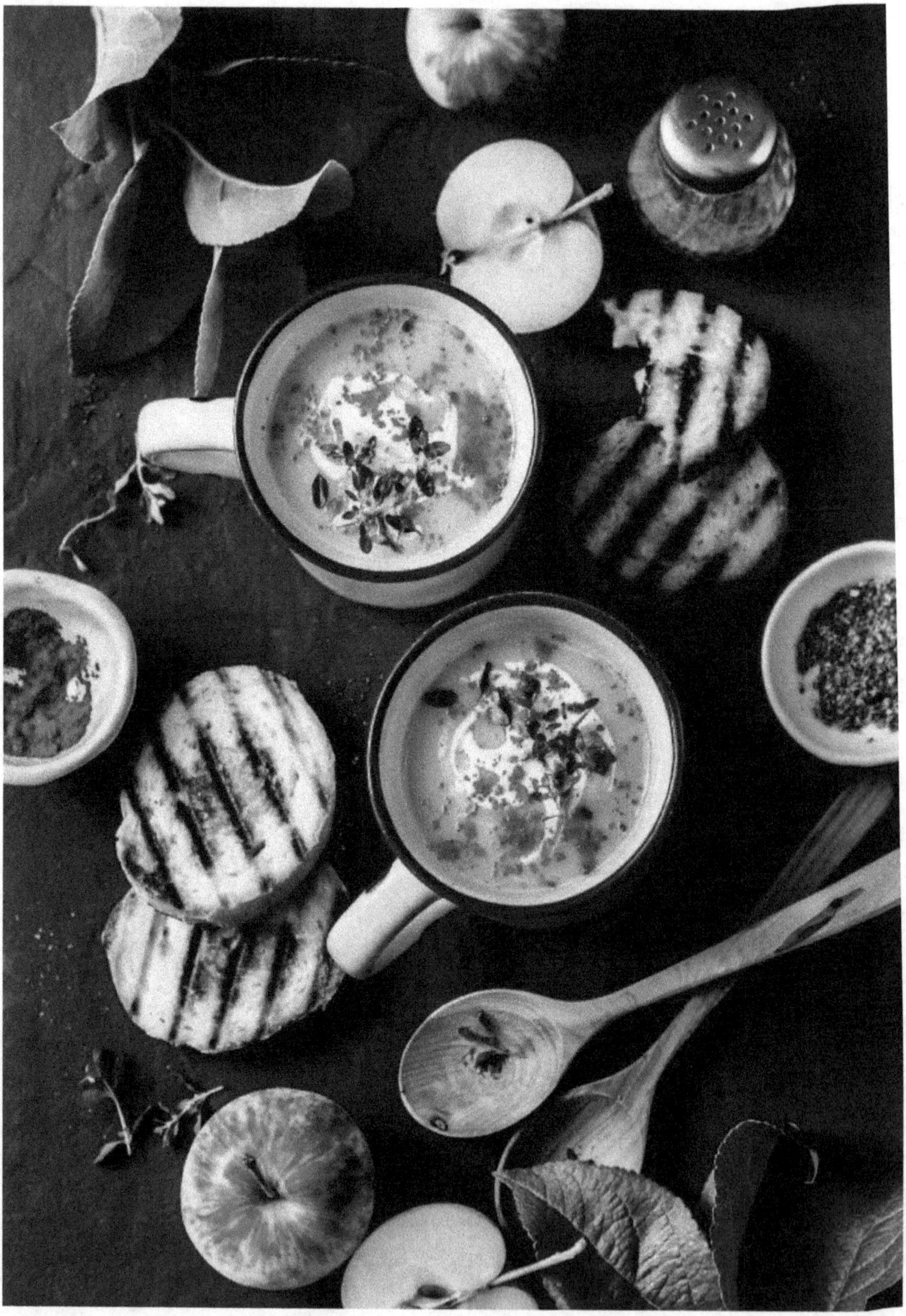

Table of Contents
Sommario

—

—

Introduction

Paleo Diet: What is it and why is it so popular?

Is the Paleo diet, an eating plan modeled after prehistoric human diets, suitable for modern humans?

A paleo diet consists of an eating plan that is based on foods similar to what might have been eaten during the Paleolithic era, which dates back about 2.5 million to 10,000 years ago.

A paleo diet generally includes lean meats, fish, fruits, vegetables, nuts, and seeds - foods that could be obtained through hunting and gathering in the past. A paleo diet places limits on foods that became common when agriculture emerged about 10,000 years ago. These foods include dairy, legumes, and grains.

Other terms for a paleo diet are paleolithic diet, stone age diet, hunter-gatherer diet, and caveman diet.

Purpose

The goal of a paleo diet is to return to a way of eating more like what primitive humans ate. The principle of the diet is that the human body is genetically unsuited to the modern diet that emerged with agricultural practices - an idea known as the dissonance hypothesis.

Agriculture changed what people ate and introduced dairy, grains, and legumes as additional staples in the human diet. This relatively late and rapid change in diet, according to the hypothesis, outpaced the body's ability to adapt. This mismatch is believed to be a contributing factor to the prevalence of obesity, diabetes, and heart disease today.

Why you might follow a paleo diet

You may decide to follow a paleo diet because:

You want to lose weight or maintain a healthy weight
You want help planning your meals

Details of a paleo diet

Indications vary among paleo diets on the market, and some diet plans have stricter guidelines than others. Usually, paleo diets adhere to these guidelines.

What to eat

Fruits

Vegetables

Nuts and seeds

Lean meats, especially grass-fed animals or wild game

Fish, especially those rich in omega-3 fatty acids, such as salmon, mackerel and albacore tuna

Oils from fruits and nuts, such as olive oil or walnut oil

What to avoid

Grains, such as wheat, oats and barley

Legumes, such as beans, lentils, peanuts and peas

Dairy products

Refined sugar

Salt

Potatoes

Highly processed foods in general

Results

Some random clinical trials have compared the paleo diet to other dietary plans, such as the Mediterranean diet or the diabetes diet. In general, these studies show that a paleo diet can provide some benefits over diets based on fruits, vegetables, lean meats, whole grains, legumes, and low-fat dairy products. These benefits may include:

Increased weight loss

Improved glucose tolerance

Improved blood pressure control

Lower triglycerides

Improved appetite management

Questions about the paleo diet hypothesis

Scientists have argued that the hypothesis behind the paleo diet may oversimplify the story of how humans adapted to changes in diet. Evidence in favor of a more complex view of the evolution of human nutritional needs includes the following:

- Changes in diet based on geography, climate, and food availability - not just the transition to agriculture - would also have shaped the evolution of nutritional needs.

- Archaeological research has shown that early human diets may have included wild grains up to 30,000 years ago - well before the introduction of agriculture.

- Genetic research has shown that significant evolutionary changes continued after the Paleolithic era, including diet-related changes such as an increase in the number of genes linked to the breakdown of dietary starches.

The bottom line

A paleo diet can help you lose weight or maintain it. It can also result in other positive health effects.

In this book, you can discover different recipes to follow a diet with the principles of the Paleo diet. Enjoy!

Turkey Jalapeno and Cauliflower Casserole

Ingredients

1 pound ground turkey

1 small cauliflower, chopped

1 cup cashew cheese, shredded

½ cups nutritional yeast, shredded 1 cup sour cream

Vegetable Ingredients

1 whole jalapeno, chopped

¼ cup chopped green bell pepper

¼ cup chopped red onion Spice Ingredients

1 tsp. Cumin

1 tsp. Cilantro Pinch of turmeric

1 tbsp. Minced garlic

Preheat the oven to 350 degrees F

Place the minced meat and cauliflower in a bowl and add the spice ingredients. Add the vegetable ingredients.

Mix in 1 cup of nutritional yeast Pour this into a casserole dish.

Top with the remaining cashew cheese and nutritional yeast. Bake for 1 hour.

Top with sour cream.

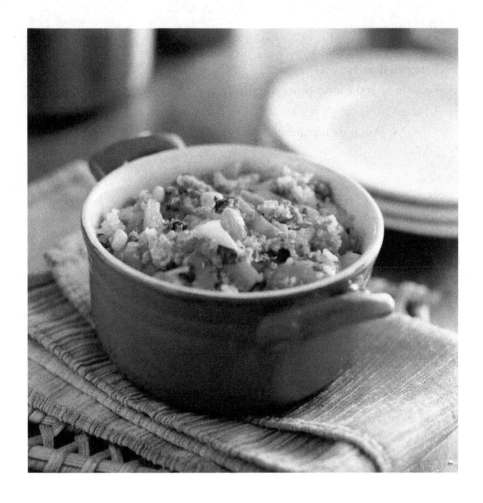

Lamb and Jalapeno Casserole

Ingredients

1 pound ground lamb

1 small cauliflower, chopped

1 cup cashew cheese, shredded

½ cups nutritional yeast, shredded 1 cup sour cream

Vegetable Ingredients

1 whole jalapeno, chopped

¼ cup chopped green bell pepper

¼ cup chopped red onion Spice Ingredients

1 tsp. Cumin

1 tsp. Cilantro Pinch of turmeric

1 tbsp. Minced garlic

Preheat the oven to 350 degrees F

Place the minced meat and cauliflower in a bowl and add the spice ingredients. Add the vegetable ingredients.

Mix in 1 cup of nutritional yeast Pour this into a casserole dish.

Top with the remaining cashew cheese and nutritional yeast. Bake for 1 hour.

Top with sour cream.

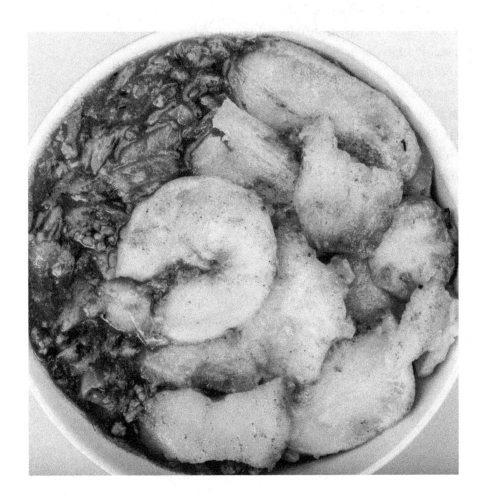

Smoky Mackerel Casserole

Ingredients
1 pound canned mackerel
1 small cauliflower, chopped
1 cup cashew cheese, shredded
½ cups nutritional yeast, shredded 1 cup sour cream
Vegetable Ingredients
1 whole jalapeno, chopped
¼ cup chopped green bell pepper
¼ cup chopped red onion Spice Ingredients
1 tsp. Cumin
1 tsp. Cilantro Pinch of turmeric
1 tbsp. Minced garlic

Preheat the oven to 350 degrees F
Place the minced fish and cauliflower in a bowl and add the spice ingredients. Add the vegetable ingredients.
Mix in 1 cup of nutritional yeast Pour this into a casserole dish.
Top with the remaining cashew cheese and nutritional yeast. Bake for 1 hour.
Top with sour cream.

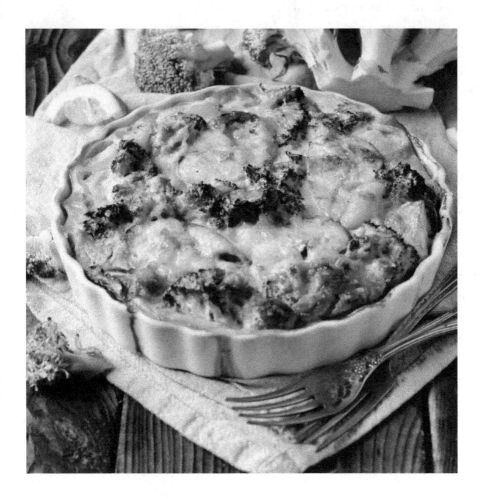

Crab Casserole

Ingredients

1 pound canned crab meat

1 small cauliflower, chopped

1 cup cashew cheese, shredded

½ cups nutritional yeast, shredded 1 cup sour cream

Vegetable Ingredients

1 whole jalapeno, chopped

¼ cup chopped green bell pepper

¼ cup chopped red onion Spice Ingredients

1 tsp. Cumin

1 tsp. Cilantro Pinch of turmeric

1 tbsp. Minced garlic

Preheat the oven to 350 degrees F

Place the crab meat and cauliflower in a bowl and add the spice ingredients. Add the vegetable ingredients.

Mix in 1 cup of nutritional yeast Pour this into a casserole dish.

Top with the remaining cashew cheese and nutritional yeast. Bake for 1 hour.

Top with sour cream.

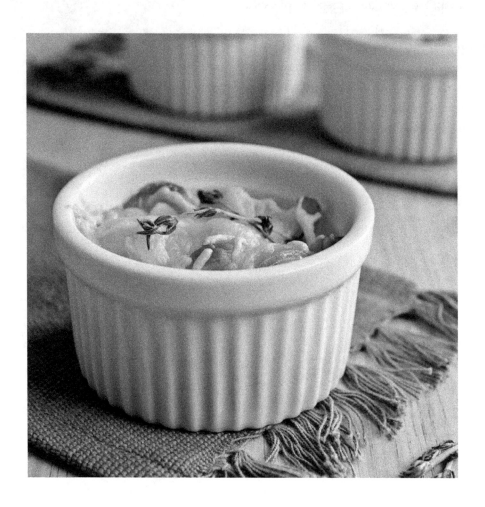

Roasted Cauliflower

Ingredients
10 medium cauliflower, sliced diagonally into chunks
¾ cup extra virgin olive oil 3 tbsp. Italian Seasoning
2 tbsp. Kosher Salt 2 tbsp. maple syrup

Preheat the oven to 170 degrees F.
Place the cauliflower in a baking pan with the cut side up.
Drizzle with 2/3 cup extra virgin olive oil, raw honey, Italian seasoning and salt. Bake for 10 hours.
Drizzle with the remaining olive oil when you serve.
Cook's Note:
Do this overnight.

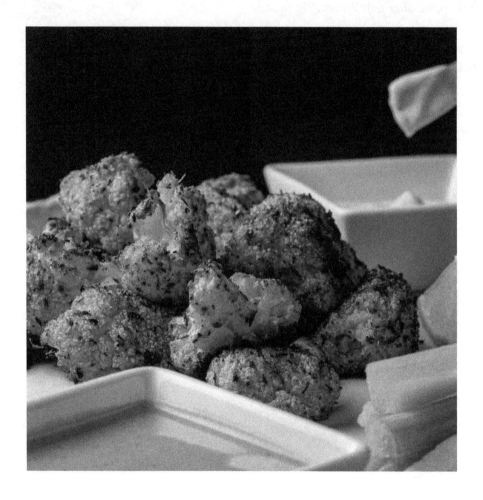

Roasted Brussel Sprouts

Ingredients
10 medium Brussel sprouts, sliced diagonally into chunks
¾ cup extra virgin olive oil 3 tbsp. Italian Seasoning
2 tbsp. Kosher Salt 2 tbsp. raw honey

Preheat the oven to 170 degrees F.
Place the Brussel sprouts in a baking pan with the cut side up.
Drizzle with 2/3 cup extra virgin olive oil, raw honey, Italian seasoning and salt. Bake for 10 hours.
Drizzle with the remaining olive oil when you serve.
Cook's Note:
Do this overnight.

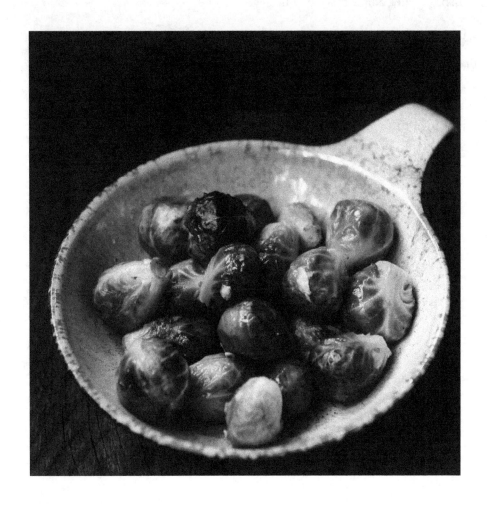

Roasted Sweet Potatoes with Raw Honey

Ingredients

10 medium sweet potatoes, sliced diagonally into chunks

¾ cup extra virgin olive oil 3 tbsp. Italian Seasoning

2 tbsp. Kosher Salt 2 tbsp. raw honey

Preheat the oven to 170 degrees F.

Place the sweet potatoes in a baking pan with the cut side up.

Drizzle with 2/3 cup extra virgin olive oil, raw honey, Italian seasoning and salt. Bake for 10 hours.

Drizzle with the remaining olive oil when you serve.

Cook's Note:

Do this overnight.

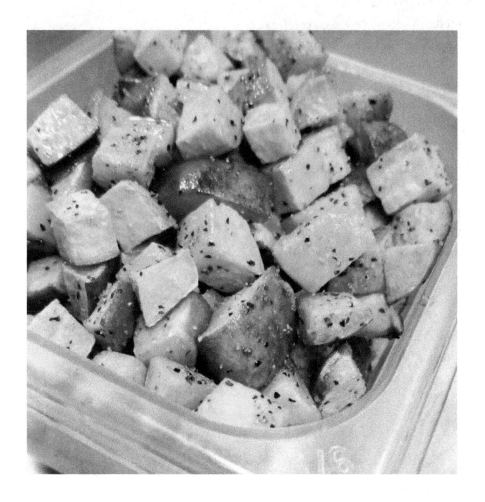

Spicy Beef and Lamb Meatballs

Main Ingredients
½ pound ground beef
½ pound ground lamb
2 medium yellow onions, chopped
½ medium yellow bell pepper 2 tbsp. Cilantro, finely chopped
½ tsp. cumin
½ tsp. chili powder
½ tsp. Sea Salt
½ tsp. Red pepper flakes
Juice and zest of ¼ medium lemon 2 ounces cashew cheese
2 tbsp. Flaxseed meal 2 tbsp. Almond flour

Guacamole
1 medium avocado
Juice of ⅓ of medium lime 1 tbsp. finely minced garlic Sea Salt
Extra virgin olive oil

Preheat the oven to 350 degrees F.
Combine all of the main ingredients together. Roll them into meatballs and bake for 18 min. Combine all of the guacamole ingredients. Serve the meatballs with guacamole.

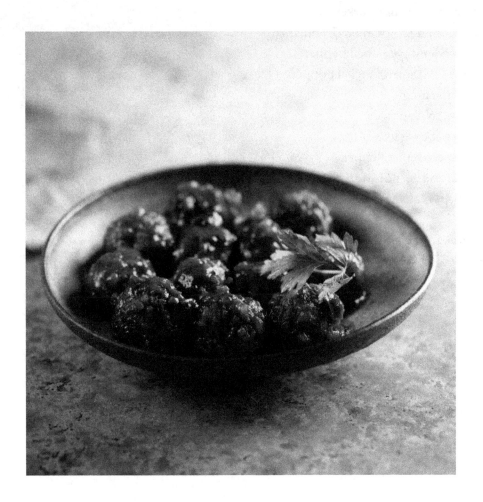

Chicken Turkey and Green Bell Pepper Meatballs

Main Ingredients
½ pound ground chicken
½ pound ground turkey
2 medium red onions, chopped
½ medium green bell pepper
2 tbsp. Cilantro, finely chopped
½ tsp. cumin
½ tsp. chili powder
½ tsp. Sea Salt
½ tsp. cayenne pepper
Juice and zest of ¼ medium lime 2 ounces cashew cheese
2 tbsp. Flaxseed meal 2 tbsp. Almond flour

Guacamole
1 medium avocado
Juice of ⅓ of medium lime 1 tbsp. finely minced garlic Sea Salt
Extra virgin olive oil

Preheat the oven to 350 degrees F.
Combine all of the main ingredients together. Roll them into meatballs and bake for 18 min. Combine all of the guacamole ingredients.
Serve the meatballs with guacamole.

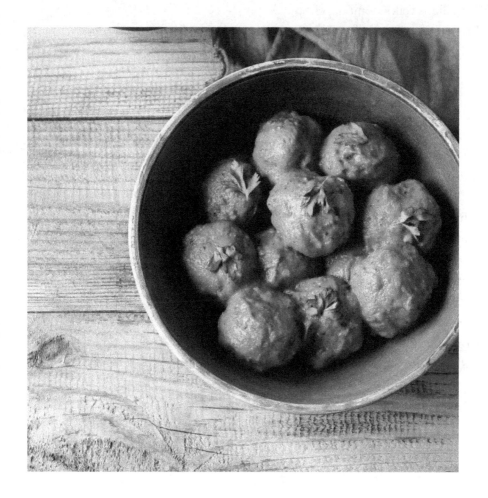

Beef Pork and Green Bell Pepper Meatballs

Main Ingredients
½ pound ground beef
½ pound ground pork
2 medium yellow onions, chopped
½ medium green bell pepper
2 tbsp. Cilantro, finely chopped
½ tsp. Onion powder
½ tsp. Cayenne pepper
½ tsp. Sea Salt
½ tsp. Red pepper flakes
Juice and zest of ¼ medium lime 2 ounces cashew cheese
2 tbsp. Flaxseed meal 2 tbsp. Almond flour

Guacamole
1 medium avocado
Juice of ⅓ of medium lime 1 tbsp. finely minced garlic Sea Salt
Extra virgin olive oil

Preheat the oven to 350 degrees F.
Combine all of the main ingredients together. Roll them into meatballs and bake for 18 min. Combine all of the guacamole ingredients.
Serve the meatballs with guacamole.

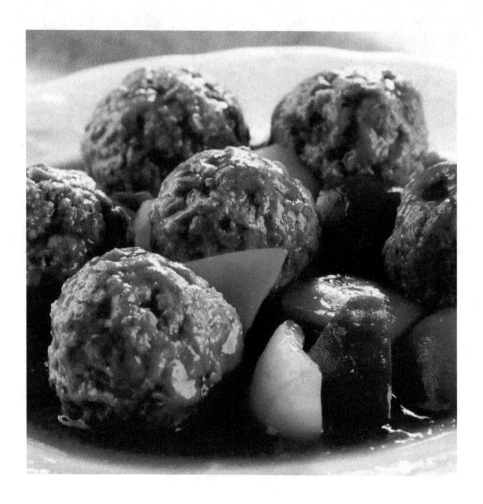

Spicy Beef Pork and Bell Pepper Meatballs

Main Ingredients
½ pound ground beef
½ pound ground pork
2 medium yellow onions, chopped
½ medium green bell pepper
2 tbsp. Cilantro, finely chopped
½ tsp. Onion powder
½ tsp. Cayenne pepper
½ tsp. Sea Salt
½ tsp. Red pepper flakes
Juice and zest of ¼ medium lime 2 ounces cashew cheese
2 tbsp. Flaxseed meal 2 tbsp. Almond flour

Guacamole
1 medium avocado
Juice of ⅓ of medium lime 1 tbsp. finely minced garlic Sea Salt
Extra virgin olive oil

Preheat the oven to 350 degrees F.
Combine all of the main ingredients together. Roll them into meatballs and bake for 18 min. Combine all of the guacamole ingredients.
Serve the meatballs with guacamole.

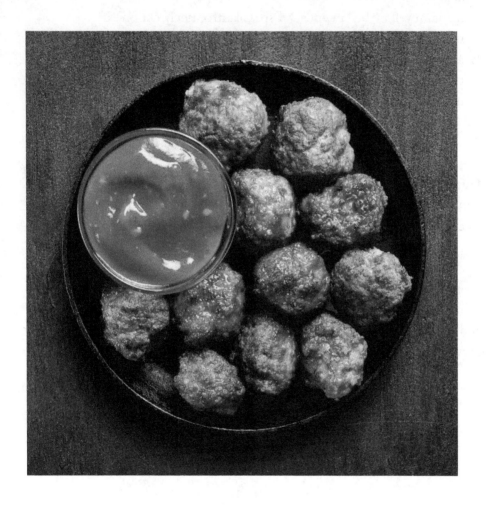

Chili Lamb and Pork Meatballs

Main Ingredients
½ pound ground lamb
½ pound ground pork
2 medium red onions, chopped
½ medium yellow bell pepper 2 tbsp. Cilantro, finely chopped
½ tsp. Onion powder
½ tsp. Chili Powder
½ tsp. Sea Salt
½ tsp. Red pepper flakes
Juice and zest of ¼ medium lemon 2 ounces cashew cheese
2 tbsp. Flaxseed meal 2 tbsp. Almond flour

Guacamole
1 medium avocado
Juice of ⅓ of medium lime 1 tbsp. finely minced garlic Sea Salt
Extra virgin olive oil

Preheat the oven to 350 degrees F.
Combine all of the main ingredients together. Roll them into meatballs
and bake for 18 min. Combine all of the guacamole ingredients.
Serve the meatballs with guacamole.

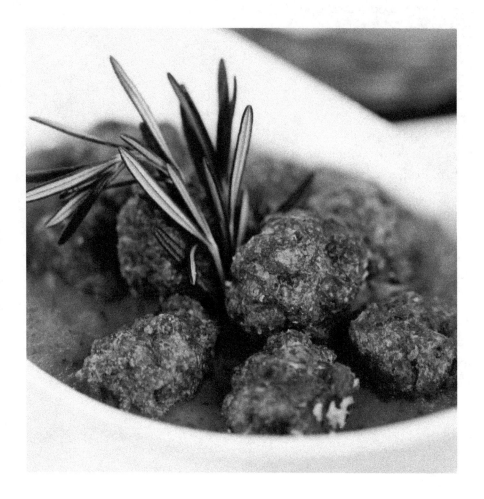

Smoky chicken Turkey and Red Onion Meatballs

Main Ingredients
½ pound ground chicken
½ pound ground turkey
2 medium red onions, chopped
½ medium green bell pepper
2 tbsp. Cilantro, finely chopped
½ tsp. cumin
½ tsp. chili powder
½ tsp. Sea Salt
½ tsp. cayenne pepper
Juice and zest of ¼ medium lime 2 ounces cashew cheese
2 tbsp. Flaxseed meal 2 tbsp. Almond flour

Guacamole
1 medium avocado
Juice of ⅓ of medium lime 1 tbsp. finely minced garlic Sea Salt
Extra virgin olive oil

Preheat the oven to 350 degrees F.
Combine all of the main ingredients together. Roll them into meatballs and bake for 18 min. Combine all of the guacamole ingredients.
Serve the meatballs with guacamole.

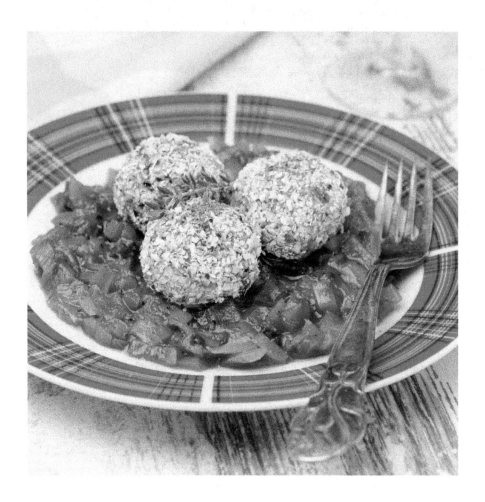

Smoky Beef Pork and Onion Meatballs

Main Ingredients
½ pound ground beef
½ pound ground pork
2 medium yellow onions, chopped
½ medium green bell pepper
2 tbsp. Cilantro, finely chopped
½ tsp. Onion powder
½ tsp. Cayenne pepper
½ tsp. Sea Salt
½ tsp. Red pepper flakes
Juice and zest of ¼ medium lime 2 ounces cashew cheese
2 tbsp. Flaxseed meal 2 tbsp. Almond flour

Guacamole
1 medium avocado
Juice of ⅓ of medium lime 1 tbsp. finely minced garlic Sea Salt
Extra virgin olive oil

Preheat the oven to 350 degrees F.
Combine all of the main ingredients together. Roll them into meatballs and bake for 18 min. Combine all of the guacamole ingredients.
Serve the meatballs with guacamole.

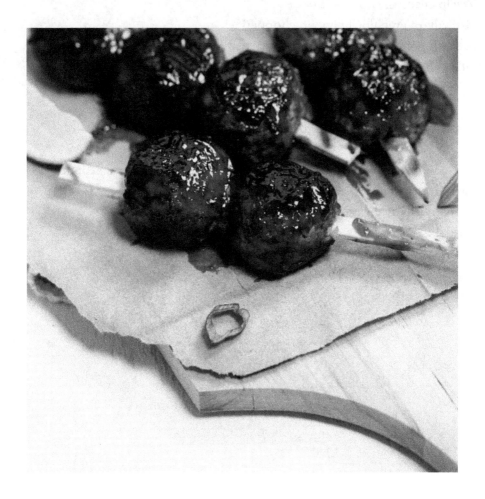

Thai Barbecue Romaine Lettuce and Bacon Salad

Salad Ingredients

4 Slices of bacon, cut into squares 2 cups romaine lettuce

¼ cup cilantro, chopped finely

¼ medium green bell pepper, chopped

Sauce Ingredients 2 tbsp. Tomato paste 3 tsp. sea salt

1 tbsp. Sesame oil 3 tbsp. Mayonnaise

½ tsp. sesame seeds

¼ tsp. assorted rainbow peppercorns 4 tsp. apple cider vinegar

½ tsp. Red pepper flakes 2 tbsp. raw honey

Over medium heat, fry the bacon until brown and crisp over medium heat. Combine the salad ingredients.

Combine all of the sauce ingredients.

Toss the salad with the sauce ingredients and top with the

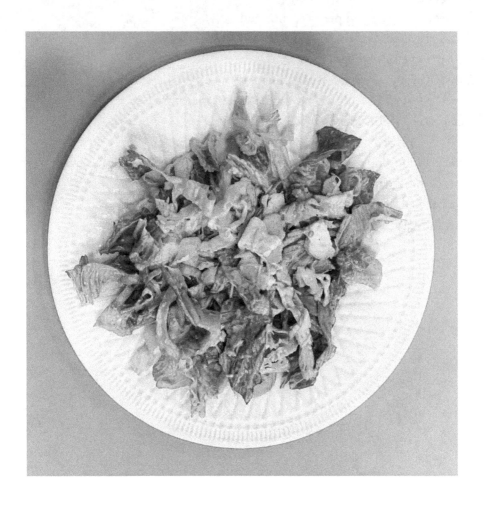

Greens and Bacon with Pesto Dressing

Salad Ingredients
4 Slices of bacon, cut into squares 2 cups loose leaf lettuce
¼ cup cilantro, chopped finely
¼ medium green bell pepper, chopped
Sauce Ingredients 2 tbsp. Tomato paste 3 tbsp. sea salt
2 tbsp. olive oil 1 tbsp. Pesto
2 tbsp. Chopped parsley 1 tsp. mustard
Juice & zest of ½ lemon 4 tsp. apple cider vinegar
½ tsp. Red pepper flakes

Over medium heat, fry the bacon until brown and crisp over medium
heat. Combine the salad ingredients.
Combine all of the sauce ingredients.
Toss the salad with the sauce ingredients and top with the bacon

Romaine Lettuce Bell Pepper and Bacon Salad

Salad Ingredients

4 Slices of bacon, cut into squares 2 cups romaine lettuce

¼ cup cilantro, chopped finely

¼ medium green bell pepper, chopped

Sauce Ingredients 2 tbsp. Tomato paste 3 tsp. sea salt

1 tbsp. Sesame oil 3 tbsp. Mayonnaise

½ tsp. sesame seeds

¼ tsp. assorted rainbow peppercorns 4 tsp. apple cider vinegar

½ tsp. Red pepper flakes 2 tbsp. raw honey

Over medium heat, fry the bacon until brown and crisp over medium heat. Combine the salad ingredients.

Combine all of the sauce ingredients.

Toss the salad with the sauce ingredients and top with the bacon

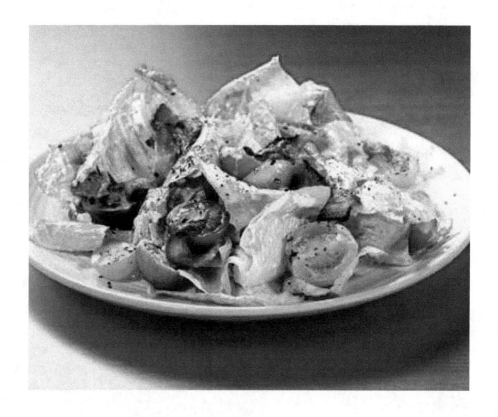

Butter head Lettuce Yellow Bell Pepper and Bacon Salad

Salad Ingredients

4 Slices of bacon, cut into squares 2 cups butter head lettuce

¼ cup cilantro, chopped finely

¼ medium yellow bell pepper, chopped

Sauce Ingredients 2 tbsp. Tomato paste 3 tsp. sea salt

1 tbsp. extra virgin olive oil 1 tbsp. Tomato sauce

2 tbsp. Chopped parsley Juice & zest of ½ lemon

¼ tsp. Sichuan peppercorns 4 tsp. white wine vinegar

½ tsp. cayenne pepper 2 tbsp. maple syrup

Over medium heat, fry the bacon until brown and crisp over medium heat. Combine the salad ingredients.

Combine all of the sauce ingredients.

Toss the salad with the sauce ingredients and top with the bacon

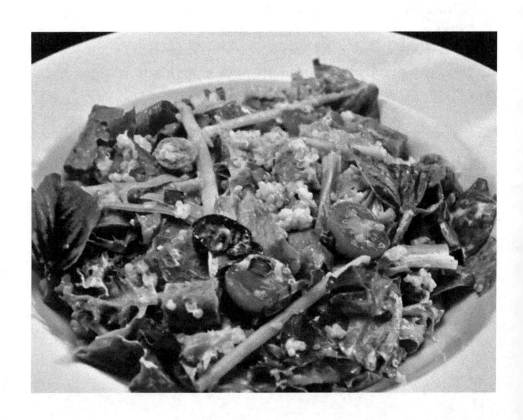

Iceberg Lettuce with Yellow Bell Pepper with Sesame Vinaigrette

Salad Ingredients
4 Slices of bacon, cut into squares 2 cups iceberg lettuce
¼ cup cilantro, chopped finely
¼ medium yellow bell pepper, chopped
Sauce Ingredients 2 tbsp. Tomato paste 3 tbsp. sea salt
1 tbsp. Sesame oil
1 tbsp. chili garlic paste 2 tbsp. Chopped cilantro
½ tsp. sesame seeds Juice & zest of ½ lime
¼ tsp. Sichuan peppercorns 4 tsp. apple cider vinegar
½ tsp. Red pepper flakes 1 tsp. Fish sauce
2 tbsp. raw honey

Over medium heat, fry the bacon until brown and crisp over medium heat. Combine the salad ingredients.
Combine all of the sauce ingredients.
Toss the salad with the sauce ingredients and top with the bacon

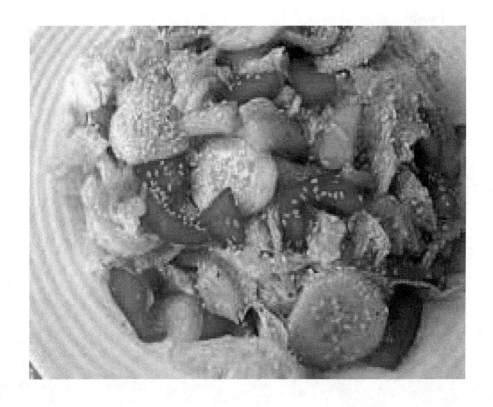

Spicy Lettuce and Bacon Salad

Salad Ingredients
4 Slices of bacon, cut into squares 2 cups loose leaf lettuce
¼ cup cilantro, chopped finely
¼ medium green bell pepper, chopped
Sauce Ingredients 2 tbsp. Tomato paste 3 tbsp. sea salt
2 tbsp. olive oil 1 tbsp. Pesto
2 tbsp. Chopped parsley 1 tsp. mustard
Juice & zest of ½ lemon 4 tsp. apple cider vinegar
½ tsp. Red pepper flakes

Over medium heat, fry the bacon until brown and crisp over medium heat. Combine the salad ingredients.
Combine all of the sauce ingredients.
Toss the salad with the sauce ingredients and top with the bacon

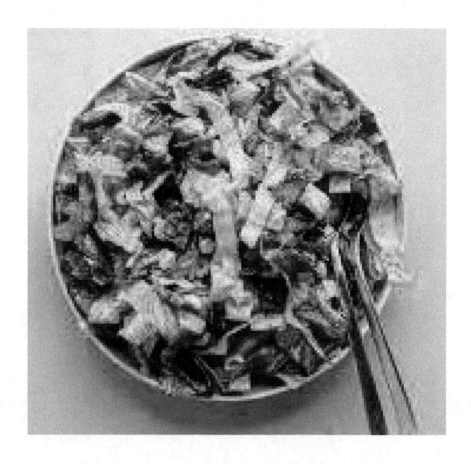

Romaine Lettuce with Green Bell Pepper with Honeyed Sesame Dressing

Salad Ingredients

4 Slices of bacon, cut into squares 2 cups romaine lettuce

¼ cup cilantro, chopped finely

¼ medium green bell pepper, chopped

Sauce Ingredients 2 tbsp. Tomato paste 3 tsp. sea salt

1 tbsp. Sesame oil 3 tbsp. Mayonnaise

½ tsp. sesame seeds

¼ tsp. assorted rainbow peppercorns 4 tsp. apple cider vinegar

½ tsp. Red pepper flakes 2 tbsp. raw honey

Over medium heat, fry the bacon until brown and crisp over medium heat. Combine the salad ingredients.

Combine all of the sauce ingredients.

Toss the salad with the sauce ingredients and top with the bacon

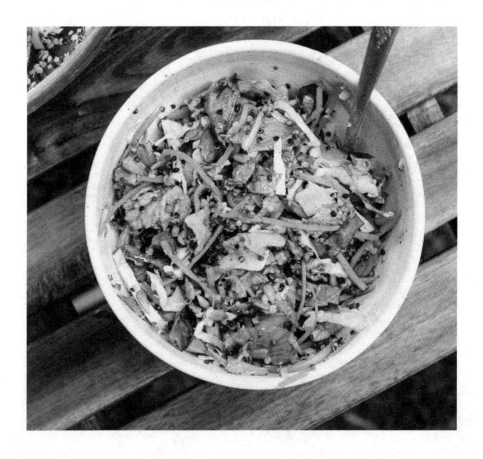

Collard Greens and Cauliflower Curry

Ingredients

Vegetable Ingredients 3/4 cup broccoli florets

1/4 cup cauliflower florets

1 large handful of collard greens 4 tbsp. Extra virgin coconut oil

¼ medium red onion

Aromatic Ingredients 1 tsp. Cilantro

1 tsp. Minced garlic 1 tsp. Minced ginger 3 tsp. Fish sauce

1 tsp. Soy sauce

½ tsp. Sea salt

1 tbsp. red curry paste 1 tbsp. Sriracha

½ cup coconut milk

Chopped onions and minced garlic

Add 2 tbsp. Coconut oil and cook over medium heat. Add onions and cook until translucent

Add the garlic and cook until golden brown. Turn the heat to medium-low and add the florets.

Keep stirring until the florets are partially cooked. Add the rest of the aromatic ingredients.

Cook for 1 more minute.

Add the remaining vegetable ingredients, coconut cream and coconut oil. Stir together and simmer for 5 to 10 min.

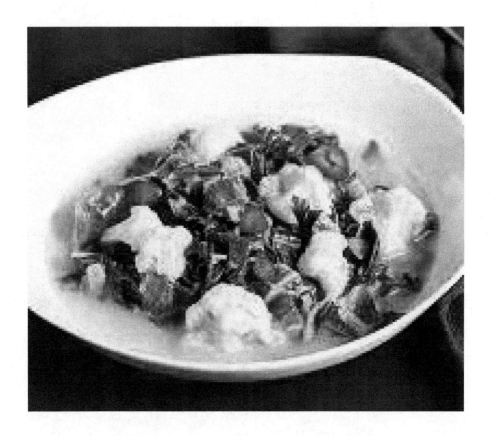

Micro greens and Cauliflower Curry

Ingredients
Vegetable Ingredients
½ cup broccoli florets
½ cup cauliflower florets
1 large handful of micro greens 4 tbsp. Extra virgin coconut oil
¼ medium onion
Aromatic Ingredients
1 tsp. Thai bird chilies, minced 1 tsp. Minced garlic
1 tsp. Minced ginger 3 tsp. Fish sauce
1 tsp. Soy sauce
½ tsp. Sea salt
1 tbsp. Green curry paste 1 tbsp. Sriracha
½ cup coconut milk
Chopped onions and minced garlic

Add 2 tbsp. Coconut oil and cook over medium heat. Add onions and cook until translucent

Add the garlic and cook until golden brown. Turn the heat to medium-low and add the florets.

Keep stirring until the florets are partially cooked. Add the rest of the aromatic ingredients.

Cook for 1 more minute.

Add the remaining vegetable ingredients, coconut cream and coconut oil. Stir together and simmer for 5 to 10 min.

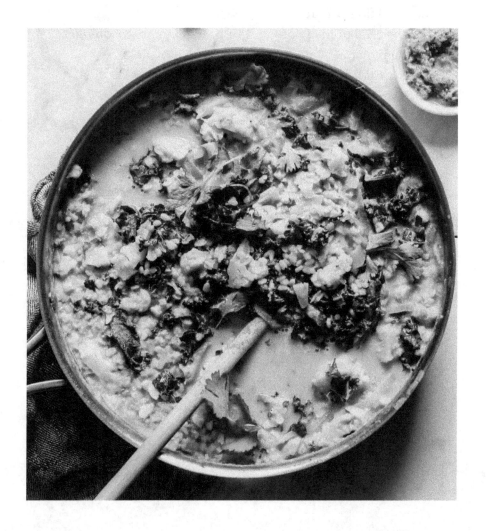

Watercress and Brussel Sprouts Curry

Ingredients
Vegetable Ingredients

½ cup brussell sprouts

½ cup cauliflower florets

1 large handful of watercress

4 tbsp. Extra virgin coconut oil

¼ medium onion

Aromatic Ingredients 1 tsp. Cayenne pepper 1 tsp. Minced garlic

1 tsp. Minced ginger 3 tsp. Fish sauce

1 tsp. Soy sauce

½ tsp. Sea salt

1 tbsp. Green curry paste 1 tbsp. Sriracha

½ cup coconut milk

Chopped onions and minced garlic

Add 2 tbsp. Coconut oil and cook over medium heat. Add onions and cook until translucent

Add the garlic and cook until golden brown. Turn the heat to medium-low and add the florets.

Keep stirring until the florets are partially cooked. Add the rest of the aromatic ingredients.

Cook for 1 more minute.

Add the remaining vegetable ingredients, coconut cream and coconut oil. Stir together and simmer for 5 to 10 min.

Micro greens and Turnip Greens Curry

Ingredients

Vegetable Ingredients

½ cup broccoli florets

½ cup turnip greens

1 large handful of micro greens 4 tbsp. Extra virgin coconut oil

¼ medium onion

Aromatic Ingredients 1 tsp. Cilantro

1 tsp. Minced garlic 1 tsp. Minced ginger 3 tsp. Fish sauce

1 tsp. Soy sauce

½ tsp. Sea salt

1 tbsp. red curry paste 1 tbsp. Sriracha

½ cup coconut milk

Chopped onions and minced garlic

Add 2 tbsp. Coconut oil and cook over medium heat. Add onions and cook until translucent

Add the garlic and cook until golden brown. Turn the heat to medium-low and add the florets.

Keep stirring until the florets are partially cooked. Add the rest of the aromatic ingredients.

Cook for 1 more minute.

Add the remaining vegetable ingredients, coconut cream and coconut oil. Stir together and simmer for 5 to 10 min.

Shrimp-Stuffed Avocado Salad

Ingredients

6 large shrimps, peeled.

6 large hard-boiled eggs, chopped

⅓ medium red onion, chopped 2 ribs of celery, chopped

¼ cup mayonnaise

2 tsp. English mustard 2 tbsp. Fresh lime juice

1 tsp. Frank's red hot sauce

½ tsp. Cumin Sea Salt

3 medium avocados

Boil the seafood until the meat is no longer translucent Combine all of the ingredients in a bowl except the avocado. Slice the avocado and take the seeds out.

Spoon the salad mixture on the avocado.

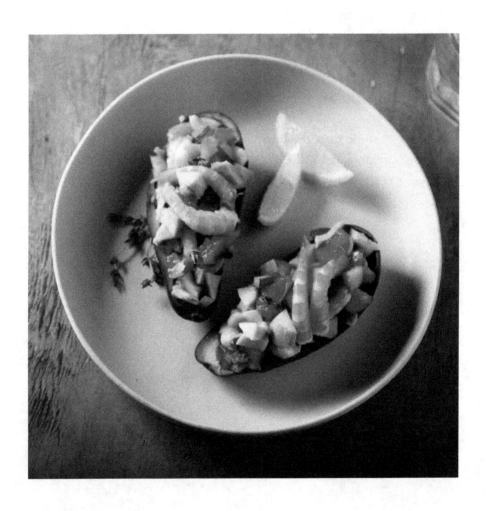

Shrimp Mango and Onion Stuffed Avocado Salad

Ingredients

6 large shrimps, peeled.

6 large hard-boiled eggs, chopped

⅓ medium yellow onion, chopped 1/2 cup cubed mangoes

¼ cup mayonnaise 2 tsp. mustard

2 tbsp. Fresh lime juice

1 tsp. Frank's red hot sauce

½ tsp. chili powder Sea Salt

3 medium avocados

Boil the seafood until the meat is no longer translucent Combine all of the ingredients in a bowl except the avocado. Slice the avocado and take the seeds out.

Spoon the salad mixture on the avocado.

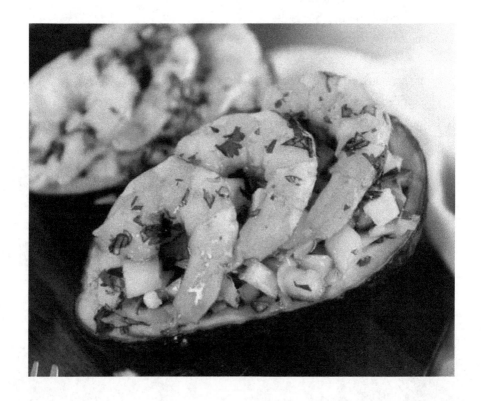

Scallop and Mango Stuffed Avocado Salad

Ingredients

7 large scallops, shells removes

6 large hard-boiled eggs, chopped

⅓ medium yellow onion, chopped 1/2 cup cubed mangoes

¼ cup mayonnaise 2 tsp. mustard

2 tbsp. Fresh lime juice 1 tsp. Tabasco hot sauce

½ tsp. Cumin Sea Salt

3 medium avocados

Boil the seafood until the meat is no longer translucent Combine all of the ingredients in a bowl except the avocado. Slice the avocado and take the seeds out.

Spoon the salad mixture on the avocado.

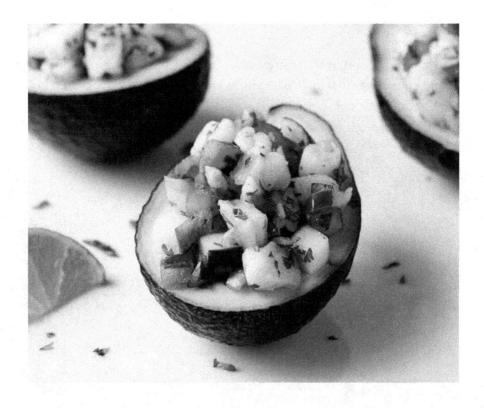

Manila Clams and Carrot Stuffed Salad

Ingredients

8 large manila clams, shells removed 6 large hard-boiled eggs, chopped

⅓ medium red onion, chopped

1/2 cup finely cubed carrots, pre-boiled

¼ cup mayonnaise 2 tsp. Dijon mustard

2 tbsp. Fresh lemon juice

1 tsp. Frank's red hot sauce

½ tsp. Cayenne pepper hot sauce

½ tsp. Cumin Sea Salt

3 medium avocados

Boil the seafood until the meat is no longer translucent Combine all of the ingredients in a bowl except the avocado. Slice the avocado and take the seeds out.

Spoon the salad mixture on the avocado.

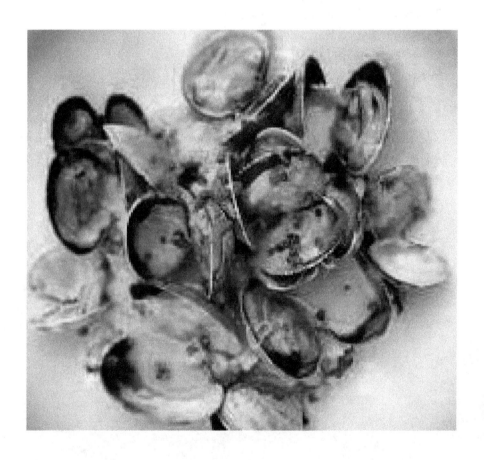

Tuna Eggs and Avocado Salad

Ingredients
1/2 cup canned tuna
6 large hard-boiled eggs, chopped
⅓ medium yellow onion, chopped 1/2 cup cubed potatoes, pre-boiled
¼ cup mayonnaise
2 tsp. English mustard
1 tbsp. Apple Cider Vinegar 1 tsp. Frank's red hot sauce
½ tsp. chili powder Sea Salt
3 medium avocados

Boil the seafood until the meat is no longer translucent Combine all of the ingredients in a bowl except the avocado. Slice the avocado and take the seeds out.
Spoon the salad mixture on the avocado.

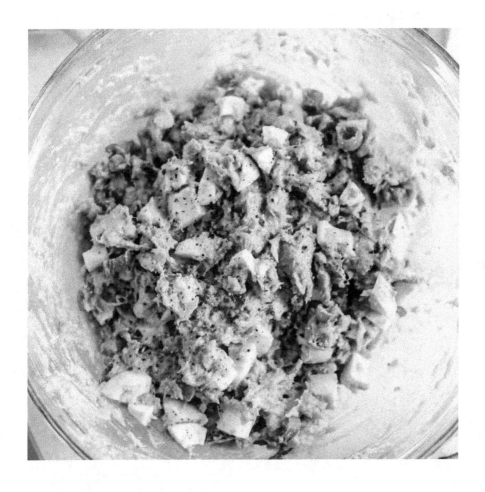

Crab and Carrot-Stuffed Avocado Salad with Spicy Lemon Dressing

Ingredients

1/2 cup canned crab meat

6 large hard-boiled eggs, chopped

⅓ medium red onion, chopped

1/2 cup finely cubed carrots, pre-boiled

¼ cup mayonnaise 2 tsp. Dijon mustard

2 tbsp. Fresh lemon juice 1 tsp. Tabasco hot sauce

½ tsp. Cumin Sea Salt

3 medium avocados

Boil the seafood until the meat is no longer translucent Combine all of the ingredients in a bowl except the avocado. Slice the avocado and take the seeds out.

Spoon the salad mixture on the avocado.

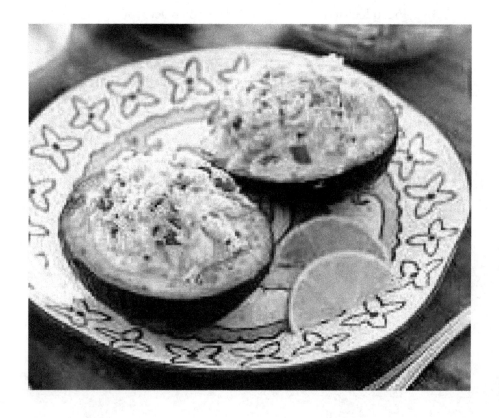

Salmon Egg and Mango-Stuffed Avocado Salad with Balsamic Dressing

Ingredients
1/2 cup canned salmon
6 large hard-boiled eggs, chopped
⅓ medium yellow onion, chopped 1/2 cup cubed mangoes
¼ cup mayonnaise
2 tsp. English mustard
1 tbsp. Balsamic Vinegar 1 tsp. Italian seasoning Sea Salt
3 medium avocados

Boil the seafood until the meat is no longer translucent Combine all of the ingredients in a bowl except the avocado. Slice the avocado and take the seeds out.
Spoon the salad mixture on the avocado.

Tilapia and Red Onion-Stuffed Avocado with Smoky Lemon Dressing

Ingredients
2 large tilapia fish fillet, cubed

6 large hard-boiled eggs, chopped

⅓ medium red onion, chopped

1/2 cup finely cubed carrots, pre-boiled

¼ cup mayonnaise 2 tsp. Dijon mustard

2 tbsp. Fresh lemon juice 1 tsp. Tabasco hot sauce

½ tsp. Cumin Sea Salt

3 medium avocados

Boil the seafood until the meat is no longer translucent Combine all of the ingredients in a bowl except the avocado. Slice the avocado and take the seeds out.

Spoon the salad mixture on the avocado.

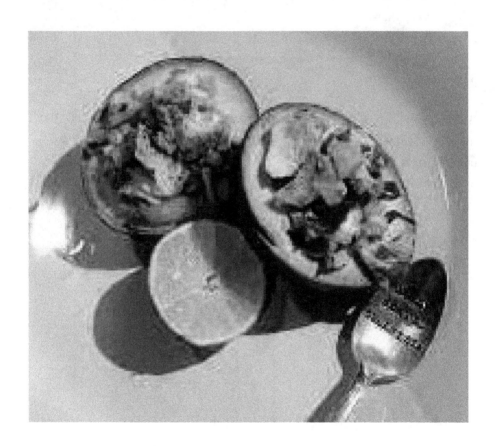

Scallop Onion and Egg-Stuffed Avocado Salad with Balsamic Dressing

Ingredients
7 large scallops, shells removes
6 large hard-boiled eggs, chopped
⅓ medium yellow onion, chopped 1/2 cup cubed mangoes
¼ cup mayonnaise
2 tsp. English mustard
1 tbsp. Balsamic Vinegar 1 tsp. Italian seasoning Sea Salt
3 medium avocados

Boil the seafood until the meat is no longer translucent Combine all of the ingredients in a bowl except the avocado. Slice the avocado and take the seeds out.
Spoon the salad mixture on the avocado.

Salmon Onion and Mango-Stuffed Avocado with Cashew Cheese

Ingredients
1/2 cup canned salmon
6 large hard-boiled eggs, chopped
⅓ medium yellow onion, chopped 1/2 cup cubed mangoes
¼ cup mayonnaise 2 tsp. mustard
1 tbsp. White Wine Vinegar 1 tsp. Cashew Cheese
½ tsp. Cumin Sea Salt
3 medium avocados

Boil the seafood until the meat is no longer translucent Combine all of the ingredients in a bowl except the avocado. Slice the avocado and take the seeds out.
Spoon the salad mixture on the avocado.

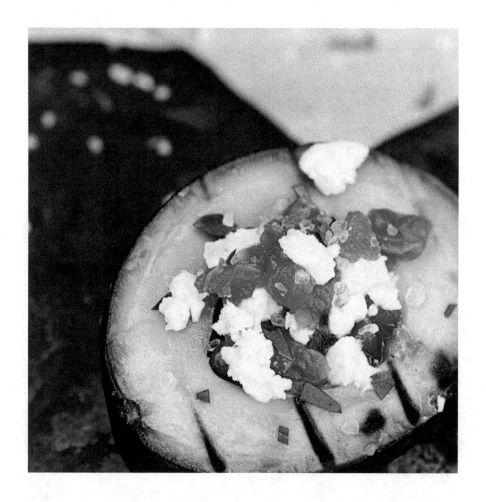

Shrimp Egg and Onion-Stuffed Avocado with Lime Dressing

Ingredients

6 large shrimps, peeled.

6 large hard-boiled eggs, chopped

⅓ medium yellow onion, chopped 1/2 cup cubed mangoes

¼ cup mayonnaise 2 tsp. mustard

2 tbsp. Fresh lime juice

1 tsp. Frank's red hot sauce

½ tsp. chili powder Sea Salt

3 medium avocados

Boil the seafood until the meat is no longer translucent Combine all of the ingredients in a bowl except the avocado. Slice the avocado and take the seeds out.

Spoon the salad mixture on the avocado.

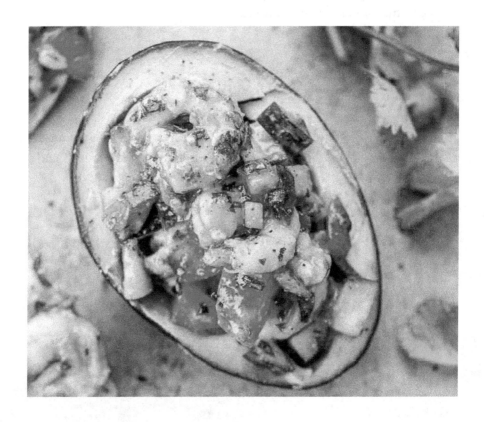

Chicken and Yellow Bell Pepper Patty

Ingredients
12 ounces chicken thigh, deboned and chopped 4 slices bacon

2 medium yellow bell peppers

¼ cup salsa

¼ cup cashew cheese 1 large egg

3 tbsp. Almond flour Pinch of sea salt

Fry the bacon until brown and crisp on medium-high heat.

In a food processor, chop the bell peppers and take out the moisture with the paper towel. Put the meat and bacon in the food processor and blend until smooth.

Add and combine this with the rest of the ingredients thoroughly.

Form into patties and fry in medium heat until golden brown.

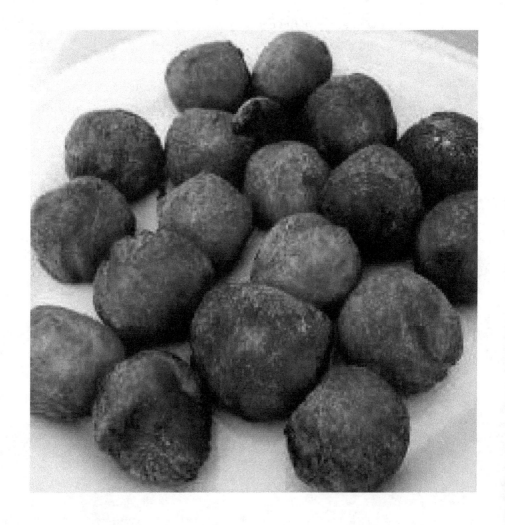

Bacon Cashew Cheese and Turkey Breast Patty

Ingredients

12 ounces turkey breast, deboned and chopped 4 slices bacon

2 medium green bell peppers

¼ cup tomatillo salsa

¼ cup cashew cheese 1 large egg

3 tbsp. Almond flour Pinch of sea salt

Fry the bacon until brown and crisp on medium-high heat.

In a food processor, chop the bell peppers and take out the moisture with the paper towel. Put the meat and bacon in the food processor and blend until smooth.

Add and combine this with the rest of the ingredients thoroughly.

Form into patties and fry in medium heat until golden brown.

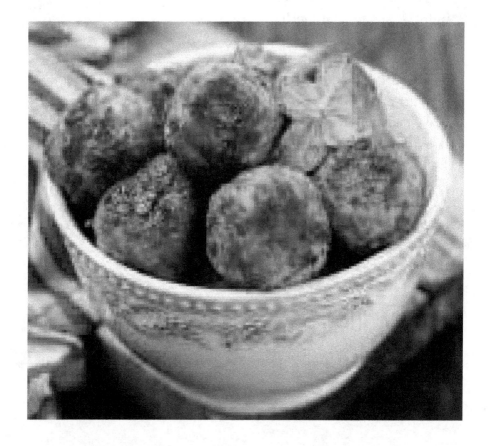

Pesto Turkey Patty

Ingredients

12 ounces turkey breast, deboned and chopped 4 slices bacon

2 medium green bell peppers

¼ cup pesto

¼ cup cashew cheese 1 large egg

3 tbsp. Almond flour Pinch of sea salt

Fry the bacon until brown and crisp on medium-high heat.

In a food processor, chop the bell peppers and take out the moisture with the paper towel. Put the meat and bacon in the food processor and blend until smooth.

Add and combine this with the rest of the ingredients thoroughly.

Form into patties and fry in medium heat until golden brown.

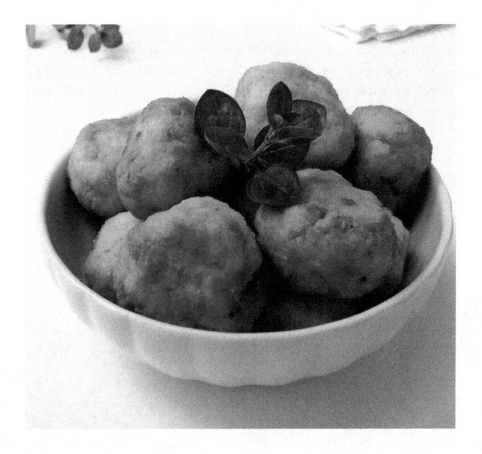

Duck and Sun-dried Tomato Pesto Patty

Ingredients

12 ounces duck breast, deboned and chopped 4 slices bacon

2 medium Sweet Italian peppers

¼ cup sun-dried tomato pesto

¼ cup nutritional yeast 1 large egg

3 tbsp. sesame seeds Pinch of sea salt

Fry the bacon until brown and crisp on medium-high heat.

In a food processor, chop the bell peppers and take out the moisture with the paper towel. Put the meat and bacon in the food processor and blend until smooth.

Add and combine this with the rest of the ingredients thoroughly.

Form into patties and fry in medium heat until golden brown.

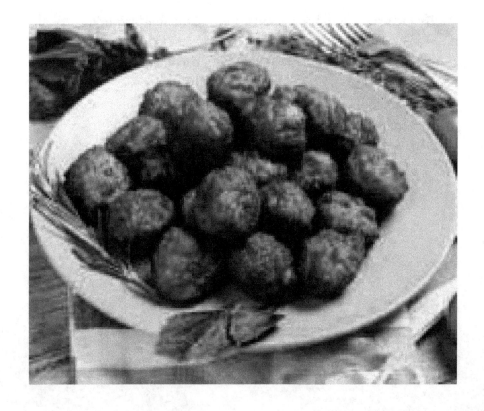

Pork Ribs and Butter Lettuce Wraps

Ingredients

5 leftover Pork Ribs

½ tsp. sesame seeds 6 pcs. Butter lettuce

⅓ Green Bell Pepper, sliced into thin strips

¼ Medium Red Onion, sliced into thin strips 2 tsp. Garlic Chili Paste

1 tsp. Sesame oil

½ tsp. sesame seeds

½ tsp. Red Pepper Flakes Sea Salt and pepper to taste

Debone the meat.

Shred the meat into small pieces.

Combine the meat with the rest of the ingredients and place them on a piece of butter lettuce. Add some salt and pepper.

Drizzle with sesame seeds Roll the lettuce up.

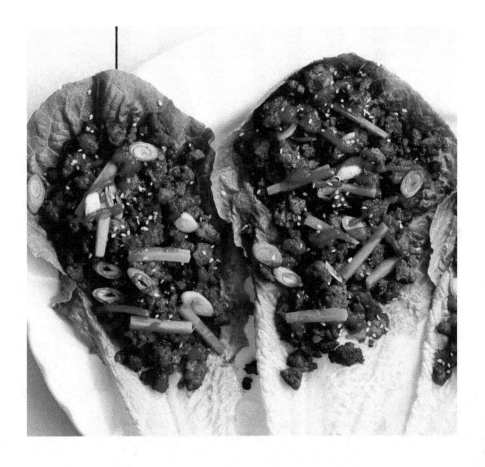

Roast Beef and Butter Lettuce Wraps

Ingredients

5 slices leftover roast beef

½ tsp. sesame seeds 6 pcs. Butter lettuce

⅓ Sweet Italian Peppers, sliced into thin strips

¼ Medium Red Onion, sliced into thin strips 2 tsp. Garlic Chili Paste

1 tbsp. almond butter 1 tsp. Peanut oil

½ tsp. sesame seeds

½ tsp. Cayenne Pepper

Sea Salt and pepper to taste

Debone the meat.

Shred the meat into small pieces.

Combine the meat with the rest of the ingredients and place them on a piece of butter lettuce. Add some salt and pepper.

Drizzle with sesame seeds Roll the lettuce up.

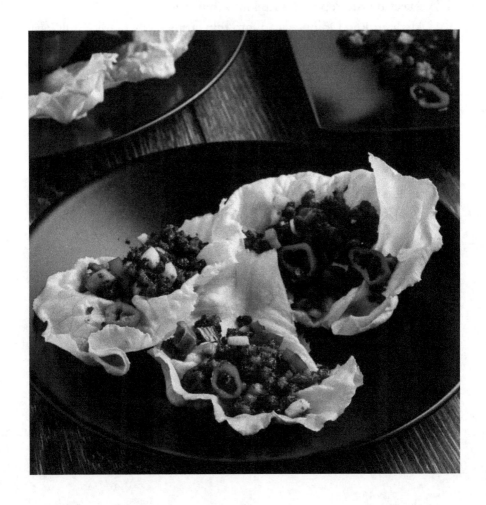

Turkey Bell Pepper and Onion Lettuce Wraps

Ingredients

half a pound leftover roast turkey

½ tsp. sesame seeds 6 pcs. Butter lettuce

⅓ Orange Bell Pepper, sliced into thin strips

¼ Medium Yellow Onion, sliced into thin strips 2 tsp. Garlic Chili Paste

1 tsp. peanut oil

½ tsp. sesame seeds

½ tsp. finely chopped spring onion Sea Salt and pepper to taste

Debone the meat.

Shred the meat into small pieces.

Combine the meat with the rest of the ingredients and place them on a piece of butter lettuce. Add some salt and pepper.

Drizzle with sesame seeds Roll the lettuce up.

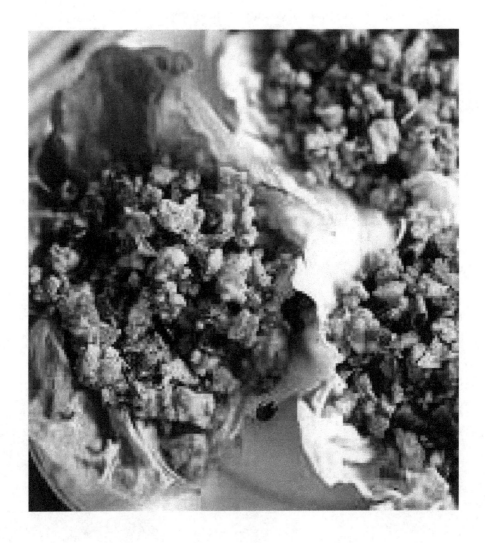

Pork Ribs Sweet Italian Peppers and Red Onion Lettuce Wraps

Ingredients

5 pcs. leftover Pork Ribs

½ tsp. sesame seeds 6 pcs. Butter lettuce

2 Sweet Italian Peppers, sliced into thin strips

¼ Medium Red Onion, sliced into thin strips 2 tsp. Tabasco Hot Sauce

1 tsp. Olive oil 3/4 tsp. sea salt 1 tsp. capers

1 tsp. kalamata olives

Sea Salt and pepper to taste

Debone the meat.

Shred the meat into small pieces.

Combine the meat with the rest of the ingredients and place them on a piece of butter lettuce. Add some salt and pepper.

Drizzle with sesame seeds Roll the lettuce up.

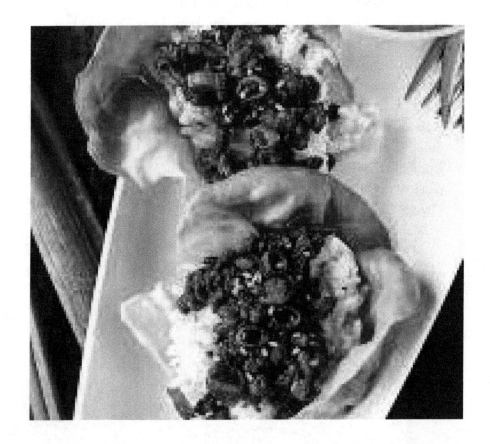

Beef Brisket Jalapeno and Red Onion Lettuce Wraps

Ingredients

10 ounces leftover barbecue beef brisket

½ tsp. sesame seeds 6 pcs. Butter lettuce

2 Jalapeno peppers, sliced into thin strips

¼ Medium Red Onion, sliced into thin strips 2 tsp. Salsa

1 tsp. Extra Virgin Olive oil 1 tsp. Red Pepper Flakes Sea Salt and pepper to taste

Debone the meat.

Shred the meat into small pieces.

Combine the meat with the rest of the ingredients and place them on a piece of butter lettuce. Add some salt and pepper.

Drizzle with sesame seeds Roll the lettuce up.

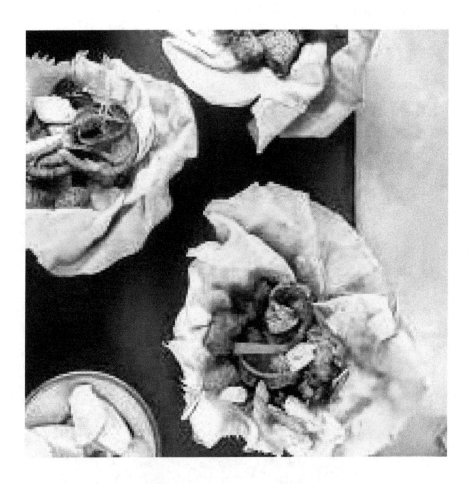

Chili Garlic Lamb Chops in Lettuce Wraps

Ingredients

3 slices of leftover lamb chops

½ tsp. sesame seeds 6 pcs. Butter lettuce

⅓ Green Bell Pepper, sliced into thin strips

¼ Medium Red Onion, sliced into thin strips 2 tsp. Garlic Chili Paste

1 tsp. Sesame oil

½ tsp. sesame seeds

½ tsp. Red Pepper Flakes Sea Salt and pepper to taste

Debone the meat.

Shred the meat into small pieces.

Combine the meat with the rest of the ingredients and place them on a piece of butter lettuce. Add some salt and pepper.

Drizzle with sesame seeds Roll the lettuce up.

Chili Garlic Roast Beef and Onion in Lettuce Wraps

Ingredients

5 slices leftover roast beef

½ tsp. sesame seeds 6 pcs. Butter lettuce

⅓ Orange Bell Pepper, sliced into thin strips

¼ Medium Yellow Onion, sliced into thin strips 2 tsp. Garlic Chili Paste

1 tsp. peanut oil

½ tsp. sesame seeds

½ tsp. finely chopped spring onion Sea Salt and pepper to taste

Debone the meat.

Shred the meat into small pieces.

Combine the meat with the rest of the ingredients and place them on a piece of butter lettuce. Add some salt and pepper.

Drizzle with sesame seeds Roll the lettuce up.

Chuck and Sirloin Burger in Portobello Bread

Ingredients

1 tbsp. Extra virgin olive oil 1 clove garlic, minced

1 tsp. Italian seasoning

¼ tsp. Sea salt

¼ tsp. Rainbow Peppercorns

2 caps Portobello mushroom caps

Burger Patty

3 ounces ground beef sirloin 3 ounces ground beef chuck 1 tbsp. English mustard

1 tsp. Sea salt.

¼ cup cashew cheese

Combine oil, salt and spices

Clean the mushrooms by taking out the gills. Marinate them with the oil and the spices

To make the patty, combine all of the burger patty ingredients. Form them into a round patty.

Place the Portobello mushrooms on the grill and cook for 8 min. Add the burger to the grill and cook for 5 min. on each side.

Top with cashew cheese.

Assemble the burger by placing it in between the Portobello mushrooms.

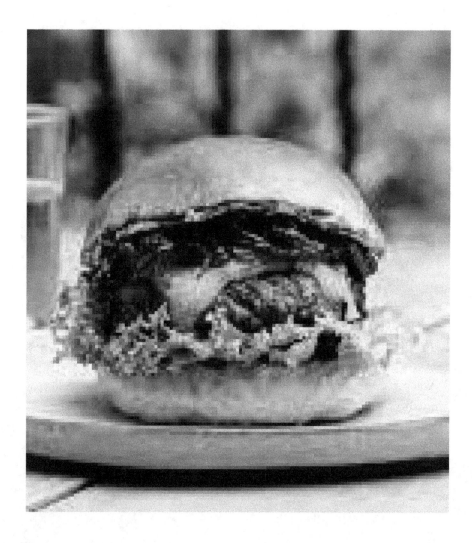

Lamb Burger in Portobello Bread

Ingredients

1 tbsp. olive oil

1 clove garlic, minced 1 tsp. Greek seasoning

¼ tsp. Sea salt

¼ tsp. Rainbow Peppercorns

2 caps Portobello mushroom caps

Burger Patty

6 ounces ground lamb 1/2 tsp. fresh rosemary 1 egg

1 tsp. Sea salt.

¼ cup cashew cheese

Combine oil, salt and spices

Clean the mushrooms by taking out the gills. Marinate them with the oil and the spices

To make the patty, combine all of the burger patty ingredients. Form them into a round patty.

Place the Portobello mushrooms on the grill and cook for 8 min. Add the burger to the grill and cook for 5 min. on each side.

Top with cashew cheese.

Assemble the burger by placing it in between the Portobello mushrooms.

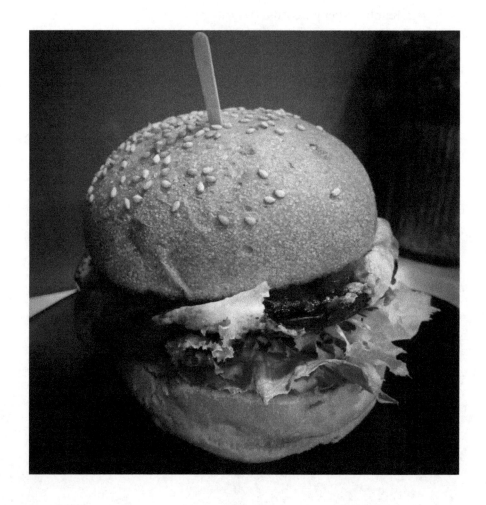

Chuck Burger in Portobello Bread

Ingredients

1 tbsp. Extra virgin olive oil 1 clove garlic, minced

1 tsp. Herbs De Provence

¼ tsp. Sea salt

¼ tsp. Black Peppercorns

2 caps Portobello mushroom caps

Burger Patty

6 ounces ground beef chuck 1 tbsp. English mustard

1 egg

1 tsp. Sea salt.

¼ cup cashew cheese

Combine oil, salt and spices

Clean the mushrooms by taking out the gills. Marinate them with the oil and the spices

To make the patty, combine all of the burger patty ingredients. Form them into a round patty.

Place the Portobello mushrooms on the grill and cook for 8 min. Add the burger to the grill and cook for 5 min. on each side.

Top with cashew cheese.

Assemble the burger by placing it in between the Portobello mushrooms

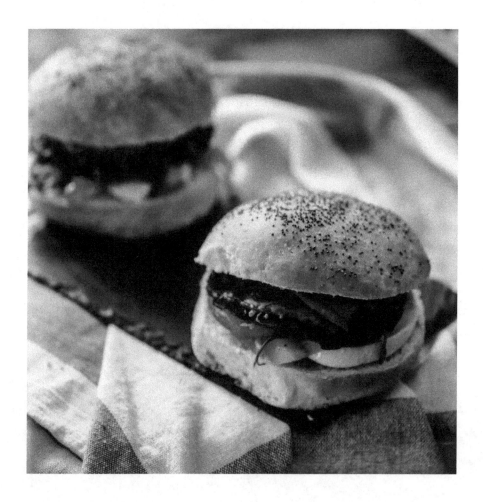

Beef Cauliflower and Cashew Cheese Casserole

Ingredients

1 pound ground beef

1 small cauliflower, chopped

1 cup cashew cheese, shredded

½ cups nutritional yeast, shredded 1 cup sour cream

Vegetable Ingredients

1 whole jalapeno, chopped

¼ cup chopped green bell pepper

¼ cup chopped red onion Spice Ingredients

1 tsp. Cumin

1 tsp. Cilantro Pinch of turmeric

1 tbsp. Minced garlic

Preheat the oven to 350 degrees F

Place the minced meat and cauliflower in a bowl and add the spice ingredients. Add the vegetable ingredients.

Mix in 1 cup of nutritional yeast Pour this into a casserole dish.

Top with the remaining cashew cheese and nutritional yeast. Bake for 1 hour.

Top with sour cream.

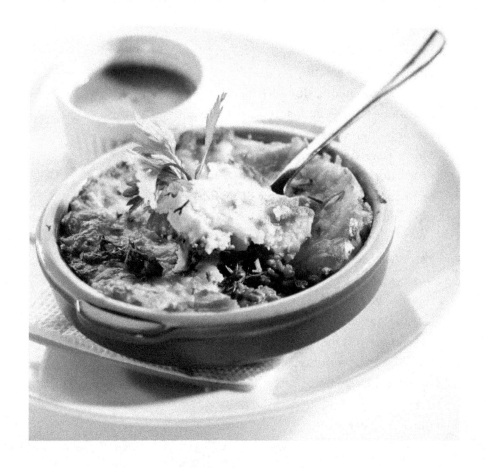

Simple Italian Roasted Carrots

Ingredients

10 medium carrots, sliced diagonally into chunks
¾ cup extra virgin olive oil 3 tbsp. Italian Seasoning
2 tbsp. Kosher Salt 2 tbsp. raw honey

Preheat the oven to 170 degrees F.
Place the carrots in a baking pan with the cut side up.
Drizzle with 2/3 cup extra virgin olive oil, raw honey, Italian seasoning and salt. Bake for 10 hours.
Drizzle with the remaining olive oil when you serve.
Cook's Note:
Do this overnight.

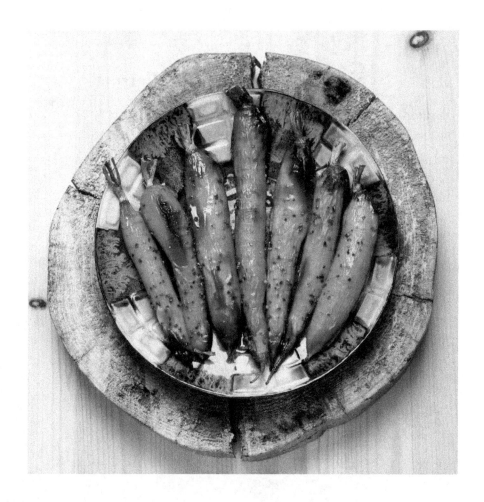

Asian Style Roasted Eggplants

Ingredients

6 medium eggplants, sliced diagonally into chunks

¾ cup sesame oil

3 tbsp. sesame seeds 2 tbsp. Sea Salt

2 tbsp. raw honey

Preheat the oven to 170 degrees F.

Place the vegetables in a baking pan with the cut side up.

Drizzle with 2/3 cup extra virgin olive oil, raw honey, Italian seasoning and salt. Bake for 10 hours.

Drizzle with the remaining olive oil when you serve.

Cook's Note:

Do this overnight.

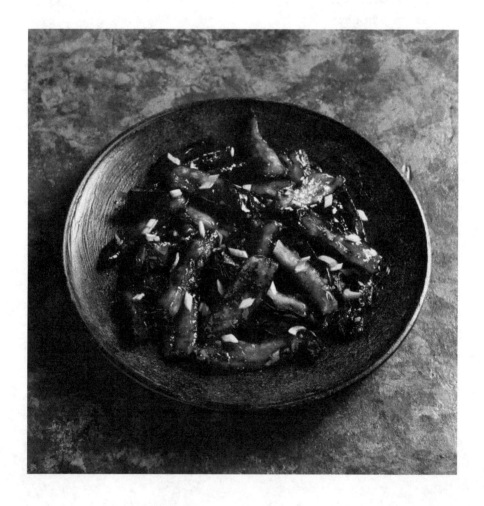

Roasted Green Bell Pepper with Bacon

Ingredients
1 1/2 pounds green bell pepper, sliced into 4 to 5 inches long strips
Olive oil, for drizzling
A few pinches black pepper 4 slices bacon
Sea salt

Preheat the oven to 400 degrees F. Lightly coat the vegetables in olive oil. Season with salt and pepper, to taste.
Divide the vegetables and wrap with bacon/pancetta.
Do this for all of the vegetables and transfer to a greased cookie sheet. Bake for 12 min.

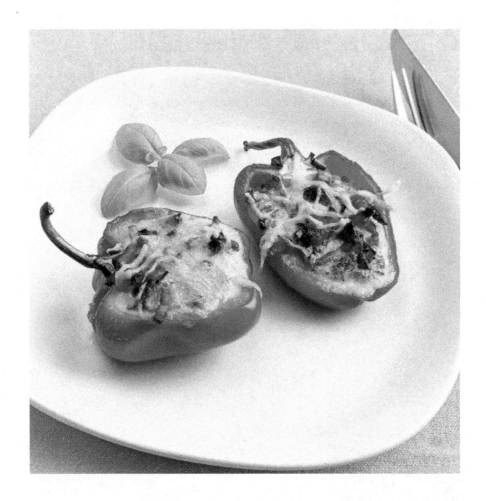

Simple Fried Calamari

Ingredients

2 pounds cleaned squid, cut into rings, see Cook's Note* 6 egg whites
2 1/2 cups almond flour Kosher salt

Add the egg whites to the almond flour and mix until smooth.
Dip the seafood into the batter and arrange them on a cookie sheet
Freeze them overnight.
Heat the deep fryer to 375 degrees F. Fry the seafood until pale gold in color. Season with salt.

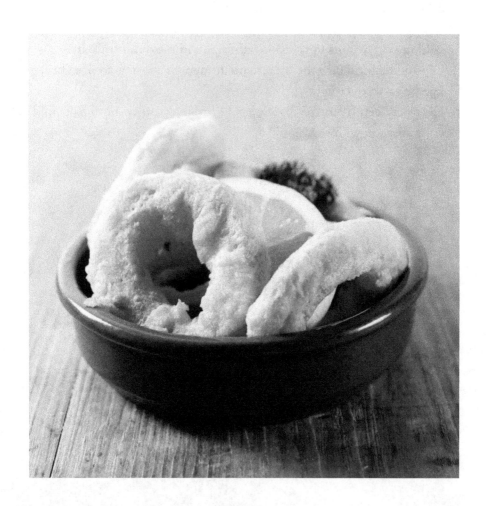

Paleo Fried Cod

Ingredients

2 pound Cod fillets or strips 6 egg whites
2 1/2 cups almond flour Kosher salt

Add the egg whites to the almond flour and mix until smooth.
Dip the seafood into the batter and arrange them on a cookie sheet
Freeze them overnight.
Heat the deep fryer to 375 degrees F. Fry the seafood until pale gold in
color. Season with salt.

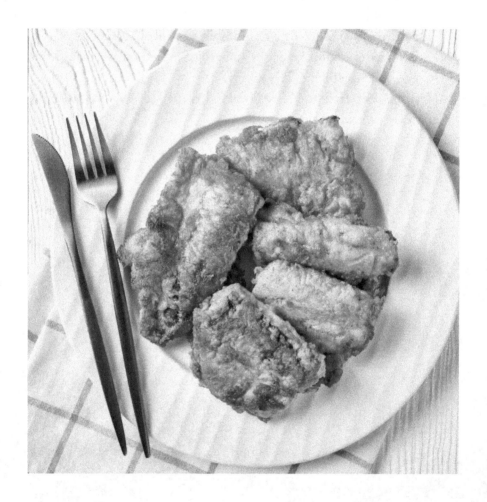

Tilapia and Green Bell Pepper Ceviche

Ingredients

2 pounds tilapia fillet 4 tomatoes, diced

5 green onions, minced 4 stalks celery, sliced

1 green bell pepper, minced 1 cup chopped fresh parsley freshly
ground black pepper

4 tablespoons extra virgin olive oil

Combine all of the ingredients and chill for one hour.

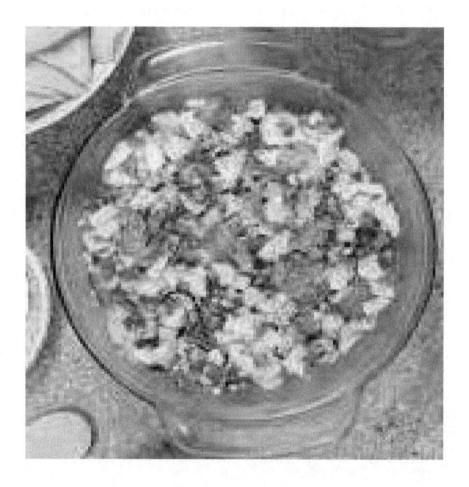

Perfectly Scrambled Eggs

Ingredients
9 Eggs
1 ½ tbsp. organic Butter, cold and cut into cubes 1 ½ tbsp. Crème fraiche
Pinch of sea salt

Break the eggs and add the butter
Stir over medium heat until it starts to cook. Remove from heat and continue stirring.
Return to the heat and continue stirring. Continue this until the butter starts to clump.
As soon as they clump, add the crème fraiche and return to the heat
Remove from heat while the eggs are soft and slightly runny and clumpy. Add sea salt to taste.

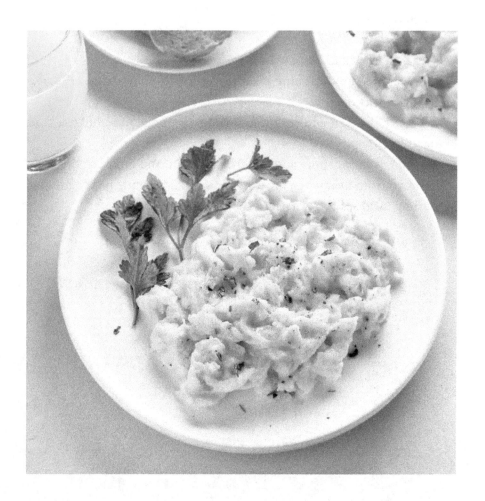

Insanely Delicious Eggs Benedict

Ingredients

4 eggs

6 slices of crisp bacon

Hollandaise sauce

½ cup wine vinegar

1 round of shallots finely sliced 6 black rainbow peppercorns

½ sprig thyme Pinch of sea salt

¾ cup butter 3 egg yolks

Juice of ¼ lemon

To make the hollandaise sauce, add vinegar, shallots, peppercorn and thyme into a pan and boil until reduced to ⅔.

Let it cool at room temperature and strain it into a bowl.

Put cubes of butter into a pan and heat until melted and foaming. Take the white foam off the surface and let it cool down to room temperature. Simmer some water in a bowl and add the yolks and the vinegar mixture.

Whisk for 9 minutes or until pale in color.

Take it out of the heat and add the melted butter and whisk until the sauce becomes creamy. If the sauce separates just add another yolk and a tbsp. of water and whisk.

Add lemon juice and salt.

Cover the bowl of hollandaise sauce.

To poach the eggs, fill the pan with water and add the vinegar and simmer. Break the eggs in a bowl.

As soon as the water simmers, stir the water in circular motion so that it swirls and add the eggs one at a time.

Take it out of the heat and let the eggs poach in the simmered water for 3 to 5 minutes. Cook the bacon in a skillet until browned.

Once the eggs are cooked, transfer to plate to dry them off. Top the bacon with eggs and drizzle with hollandaise sauce.

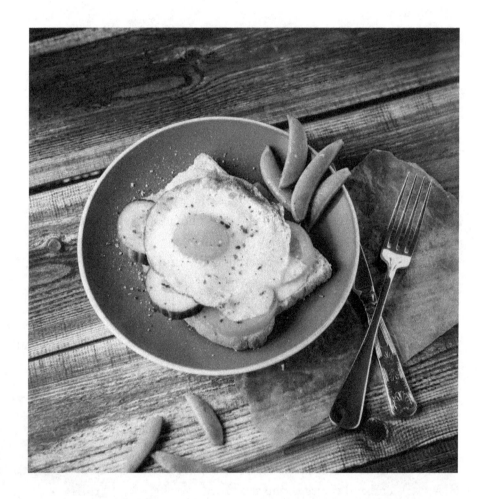

Cauliflower Turnip and Eggplant Stuffed Avocado

Ingredients

½ medium avocado 3 large eggs

Pinch of kosher salt

1 tbsp. Sliced jalapenos 4 tbsp. Nutritional Yeast 3 tsp. Tajin seasoning

1 tbsp. Extra virgin olive oil Spice Ingredients

1 tsp. Greek seasoning 1 tsp. Onion powder

½ tsp. garlic powder

¼ cup cashew cheese Filling Ingredients

3 ounces chopped cauliflower 3 ounces turnips, riced

5 ounces eggplant diced

1/2 medium green bell pepper diced Preheat the oven to 400 degrees F.

Spread all of the filling ingredients and drizzle with olive oil.

Add all of the seasoning ingredients except the cashew cheese and toss to coat. Layer evenly.

Bake for 10 to 15 min. until browned.

Take the vegetables out and top with the cashew cheese. Sliced the avocado in half and take out the seed.

Place the vegetables inside the pit of the avocado.

Add the vegetable mixture and crack the eggs on top of the mixture. Bake for 10 min.

Top with jalapenos, cashew cheese and tajin.

Broccoli Carrots and Yellow Bell Pepper Stuffed Avocado

Ingredients

½ medium avocado 3 large eggs

Pinch of sea salt

1 tbsp. Sliced jalapenos 4 tbsp. Nutritional Yeast 3 tsp. Tajin seasoning

1 tbsp. Extra virgin olive oil Spice Ingredients

1/2 tsp. cayenne pepper 1/2 tsp. herbs de Provence 1 tsp. Onion powder

½ tsp. garlic powder

¼ cup cashew cheese Filling Ingredients

3 ounces chopped broccoli 3 ounces carrots, diced

5 ounces Zucchini diced

1/2 medium yellow bell pepper diced

Preheat the oven to 400 degrees

Spread all of the filling ingredients and drizzle with olive oil.

Add all of the seasoning ingredients except the cashew cheese and toss to coat. Layer evenly.

Bake for 10 to 15 min. until browned.

Take the vegetables out and top with the cashew cheese. Sliced the avocado in half and take out the seed.

Place the vegetables inside the pit of the avocado.

Add the vegetable mixture and crack the eggs on top of the mixture.

Bake for 10 min.

Top with jalapenos, cashew cheese and tajin.

Thai Paleo Omelets

Ingredients
2 large eggs
¼ tsp. lime juice
¼ tsp. vinegar
1 tsp. Thai fish sauce 1 tbsp. Water
1 tbsp. coconut flour
1 cup extra virgin olive oil Sea salt to taste

Beat the eggs, lime juice, vinegar, fish sauce, water and coconut flour with a fork. Make sure there are no lumps.
Heat the oil over medium high heat and pour the mixture into the pan.
The egg mixture will become puffy but leave it alone.
Flip after 20 seconds.
Take the omelet out of the heat. Add sea salt to taste.

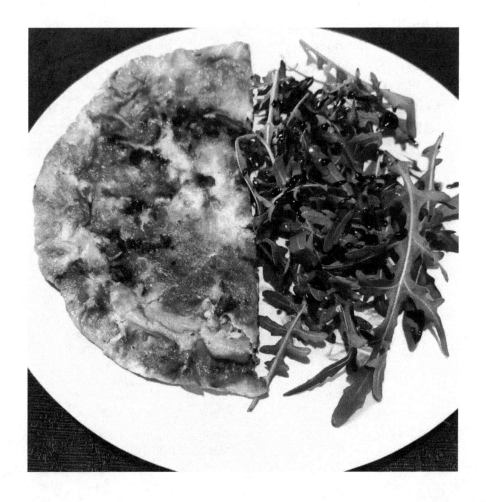

Creamy Coconut Scrambled Eggs

Ingredients

4 eggs

2-4 tbsp. coconut milk Fine sea salt, to taste

Prep

In a mixing bowl combine the eggs and coconut milk with a fork.

Cook

Melt the butter over medium low heat until bubbling. Stir salt into the egg mixture then pour into the pan. Stir slowly with rubber spatula. Once curbs begin to form turn the heat to high, fold the eggs over themselves and shake the pan constantly.

Once there's no more liquid running around the bottom of the pan, transfer it to a plate to avoid overcooking it.

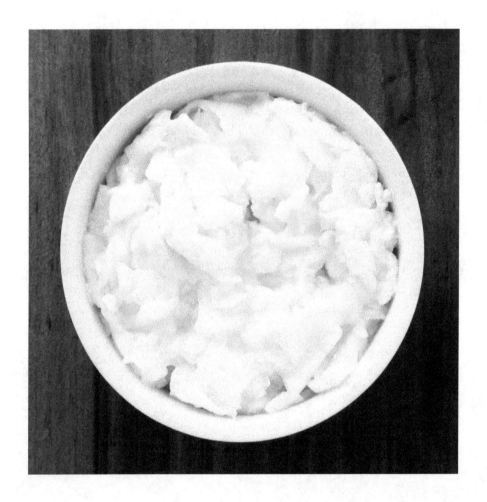

Paleo Pan-fried Chops with Caramelized Onion

Ingredients

1 tbsp. Extra virgin olive oil
4 pcs. Of 4-ounce ½-inch thick pork loin chop 1 onion cut into strips
1 cup water

Seasoning mixture
½ tsp. Sea salt
½ tsp. Paprika
½ tsp. Garlic powder
¼ tsp. Onion powder

Combine all of the ingredients for the seasoning mixture. Rub it all over the meat.

Heat a skillet in medium high heat. Brown the meat while flipping it often. Add the onions and water to the pan.

Reduce the heat and simmer for 20 min.

Turn the meat and cook until water evaporates and onions turn light to medium brown. Remove the meat and top with the onions.

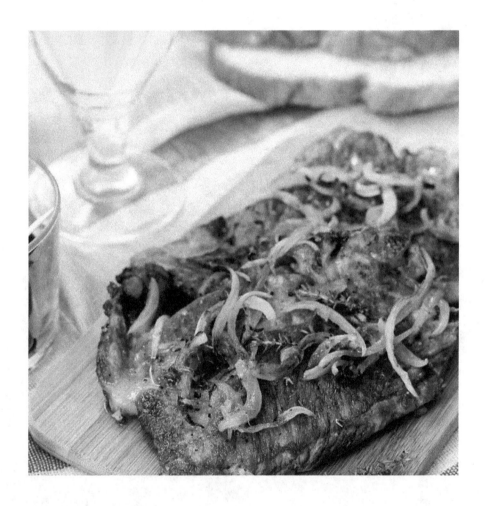

Italian Style Pan-fried Beef Tenderloin

Ingredients

1 tbsp. Extra virgin olive oil

4 pcs. Of 4-ounce ½-inch thick beef tenderloin 1 onion cut into strips

1 cup water

Seasoning mixture

½ tsp. Sea salt

½ tsp. Italian Seasoning

½ tsp. Garlic powder

¼ tsp. Onion powder

Combine all of the ingredients for the seasoning mixture. Rub it all over the meat.

Heat a skillet in medium high heat. Brown the meat while flipping it often. Add the onions and water to the pan.

Reduce the heat and simmer for 20 min.

Turn the meat and cook until water evaporates and onions turn light to medium brown. Remove the meat and top with the onions.

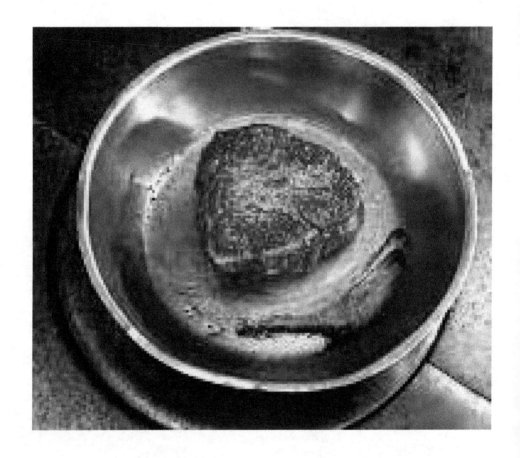

Pan-seared Halibut Fillet

Ingredients
1 tbsp. Extra virgin olive oil
4 pcs. Of 4-ounce ½-inch thick Halibut fillets 1 onion cut into strips
1 cup water

Seasoning mixture
½ tsp. Sea salt
½ tsp. Old Bay Seasoning
½ tsp. Garlic powder
¼ tsp. Onion powder

Combine all of the ingredients for the seasoning mixture. Rub it all over the fish.

Heat a skillet in medium high heat.

Sear the fish/seafood while flipping it often. Add the onions and water to the pan.

Reduce the heat to low and simmer for 12 min.

Turn the fish/seafood and cook until water evaporates and onions turn light to medium brown. Remove the fish/seafood and top with the onions.

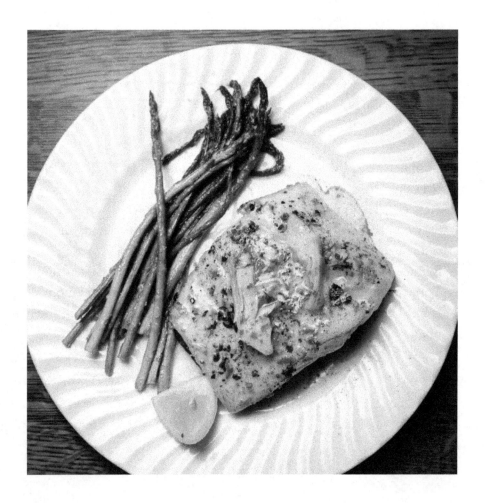

Pan-Seared Rainbow Trout Fillet

Ingredients

1 tbsp. Extra virgin olive oil

4 pcs. Of 4-ounce ½-inch thick Rainbow trout fillets 1 onion cut into strips

1 cup water

Seasoning mixture

½ tsp. Sea salt

½ tsp. Chili Powder

½ tsp. Garlic powder

¼ tsp. Onion powder

Combine all of the ingredients for the seasoning mixture. Rub it all over the fish.

Heat a skillet in medium high heat.

Sear the fish/seafood while flipping it often. Add the onions and water to the pan.

Reduce the heat to low and simmer for 12 min.

Turn the fish/seafood and cook until water evaporates and onions turn light to medium brown. Remove the fish/seafood and top with the onions.

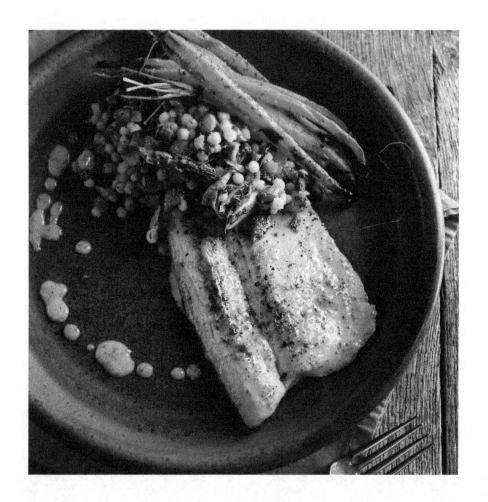

Roasted Tenderloin with Rosemary

Ingredients
4 slices 1-inch thick tenderloin roast
¼ cup extra virgin olive oil 2 tsp. Salt
Spice Ingredients
1 tsp. Herbs de Provence 1/4 tsp. Rosemary

Preheat the oven to 400 degrees F
Grease the baking sheet and rub each meat with oil.
Combine the spice ingredients and season all sides of the meat with this mixture.
Place the meat in the baking sheet and bake for 18 min. or until it reaches an internal temperature of 145 degrees F.
Notes: Make sure to take them out at 145 degrees F so you don't lose too much moisture.

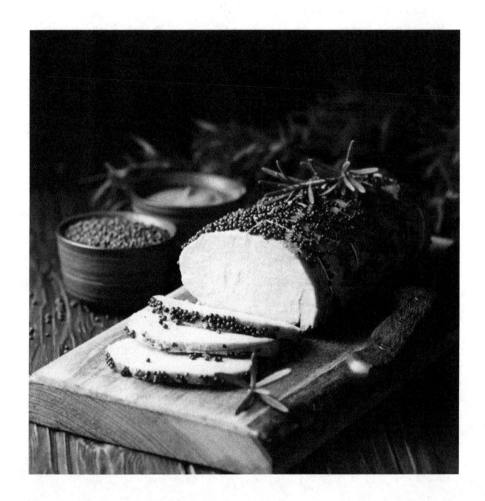

Roasted Herring Fillet with French Herb

Ingredients

4 slices 1-inch thick Herring fillets or strips

¼ cup extra virgin olive oil 2 tsp. Salt

Spice Ingredients

1 tsp. Garlic powder 1 tsp. Onion powder

1 tsp. Herbs de Provence

Preheat the oven to 400 degrees F

Grease the baking sheet and rub each fish with oil.

Combine the spice ingredients and season all sides of the fish with this mixture.

Place the fish in the baking sheet and bake for 18 min. or until it reaches an internal temperature of 145 degrees F.

Notes: Make sure to take them out at 145 degrees F so you don't lose too much moisture.

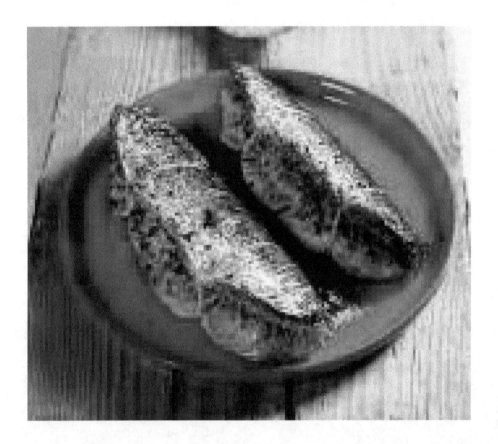

Greek Style Baked trout Fillet

Ingredients

4 slices 1-inch thick Trout fillets

¼ cup extra virgin olive oil 2 tsp. Salt

Spice Ingredients

1 tsp. Garlic powder 1 tsp. Onion powder

1 tsp. Greek Seasoning

Preheat the oven to 400 degrees F

Grease the baking sheet and rub each fish with oil.

Combine the spice ingredients and season all sides of the fish with this mixture.

Place the fish in the baking sheet and bake for 18 min. or until it reaches an internal temperature of 145 degrees F.

Notes: Make sure to take them out at 145 degrees F so you don't lose too much moisture.

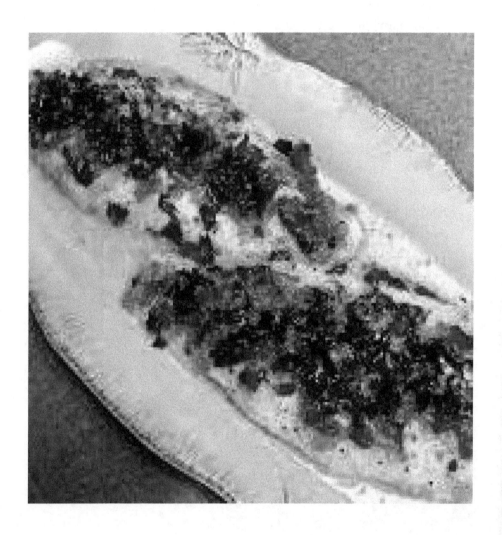

Beef Rib eye Stuffed Zucchini

Ingredients
2 large zucchini 4 tbsp. olive oil
3 ounces nutritional yeast, shredded 1 cup broccoli florets
6 ounces beef rib eye, sliced thinly
2 tbsp. Sour cream/ dairy free sour cream 1 stalk green onion
Sea salt, to taste

Preheat the oven to 400 degrees F
Cut the zucchini/eggplant lengthwise and use a melon baller to scoop
out the middle.
Pour 1 tbsp. oil into each zucchini/eggplant and season with salt and
pepper and bake for 20 min. Stir fry the meat on medium high heat.
Stir often until browned.
Cut the florets into small pieces.
Blanch the florets by dipping them into boiling water for 2 min.
Combine the florets and meat with the sour cream.
As the zucchini/eggplant finishes baking, add the meat and vegetable
filling.
Sprinkle the nutritional yeast and bake for 10 to 15 min. or until the
nutritional yeast browns. Garnish with the finely chopped green onion.

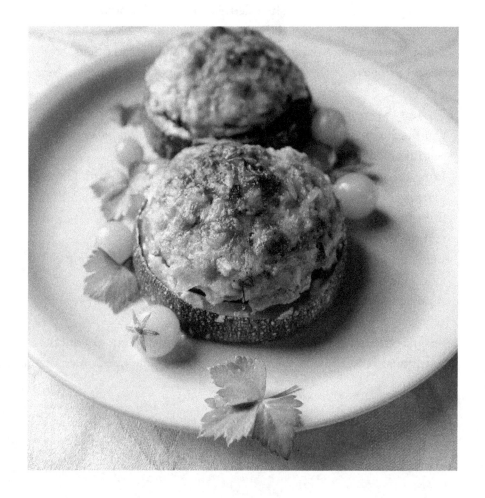

Pork Loin and Broccoli Stuffed Zucchini

Ingredients

2 large zucchini

4 tbsp. Sesame oil

3 ounces nutritional yeast, shredded 1 cup broccoli florets

6 ounces pork loin, sliced thinly

2 tbsp. Sour cream/ dairy free sour cream 1 stalk green onion

Sea salt, to taste

Preheat the oven to 400 degrees F

Cut the zucchini/eggplant lengthwise and use a melon baller to scoop out the middle.

Pour 1 tbsp. oil into each zucchini/eggplant and season with salt and pepper and bake for 20 min. Stir fry the meat on medium high heat. Stir often until browned.

Cut the florets into small pieces.

Blanch the florets by dipping them into boiling water for 2 min.

Combine the florets and meat with the sour cream.

As the zucchini/eggplant finishes baking, add the meat and vegetable filling.

Sprinkle the nutritional yeast and bake for 10 to 15 min. or until the nutritional yeast browns. Garnish with the finely chopped green onion.

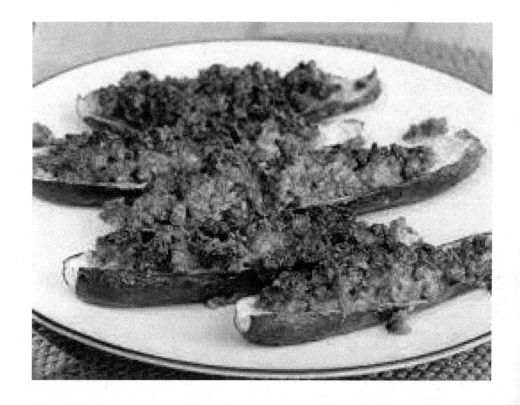

Duck Breast and Cauliflower Stuffed Zucchini

Ingredients
2 large zucchini
4 tbsp. Sesame oil
3 ounces nutritional yeast, shredded 1 cup cauliflower florets
6 ounces duck breast fillet, sliced thinly 2 tbsp. Sour cream/ dairy free
sour cream 1 stalk green onion
Sea salt, to taste

Preheat the oven to 400 degrees F
Cut the zucchini/eggplant lengthwise and use a melon baller to scoop
out the middle.
Pour 1 tbsp. oil into each zucchini/eggplant and season with salt and
pepper and bake for 20 min. Stir fry the meat on medium high heat.
Stir often until browned.
Cut the florets into small pieces.
Blanch the florets by dipping them into boiling water for 2 min.
Combine the florets and meat with the sour cream.
As the zucchini/eggplant finishes baking, add the meat and vegetable
filling.
Sprinkle the nutritional yeast and bake for 10 to 15 min. or until the
nutritional yeast browns. Garnish with the finely chopped green onion.

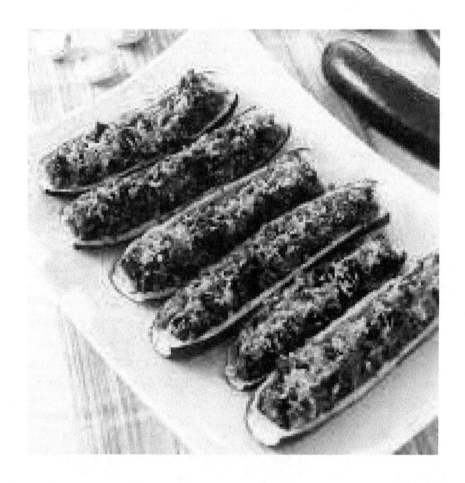

Chicken Breast and Green Onion Stuffed Eggplants

Ingredients

2 large eggplants 4 tbsp. olive oil

3 ounces nutritional yeast, shredded 1 cup cauliflower florets

6 ounces chicken breast fillet, sliced thinly 2 tbsp. Sour cream/ dairy free sour cream 1 stalk green onion

Sea salt, to taste

Preheat the oven to 400 degrees F

Cut the zucchini/eggplant lengthwise and use a melon baller to scoop out the middle.

Pour 1 tbsp. oil into each zucchini/eggplant and season with salt and pepper and bake for 20 min. Stir fry the meat on medium high heat. Stir often until browned.

Cut the florets into small pieces.

Blanch the florets by dipping them into boiling water for 2 min.

Combine the florets and meat with the sour cream.

As the zucchini/eggplant finishes baking, add the meat and vegetable filling.

Sprinkle the nutritional yeast and bake for 10 to 15 min. or until the nutritional yeast browns. Garnish with the finely chopped green onion.

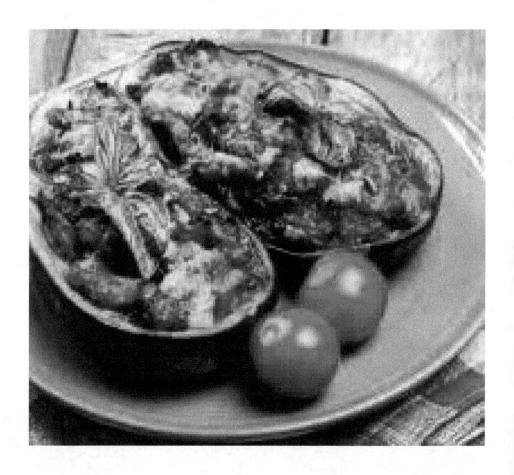

Asian Style Rib eye and Broccoli Stuffed Eggplants

Ingredients

2 large eggplants 4 tbsp. Sesame oil

3 ounces nutritional yeast, shredded 1 cup broccoli florets

6 ounces beef rib eye, sliced thinly

2 tbsp. Sour cream/ dairy free sour cream 1 stalk green onion

Sea salt, to taste

Preheat the oven to 400 degrees F

Cut the zucchini/eggplant lengthwise and use a melon baller to scoop out the middle.

Pour 1 tbsp. oil into each zucchini/eggplant and season with salt and pepper and bake for 20 min. Stir fry the meat on medium high heat. Stir often until browned.

Cut the florets into small pieces.

Blanch the florets by dipping them into boiling water for 2 min.

Combine the florets and meat with the sour cream.

As the zucchini/eggplant finishes baking, add the meat and vegetable filling.

Sprinkle the nutritional yeast and bake for 10 to 15 min. or until the nutritional yeast browns. Garnish with the finely chopped green onion.

Ice Berg Lettuce with Greek Dressing

Base Salad Ingredients
2 ¼ oz Iceberg Lettuce 1/4 cup walnuts
2   slices of bacon
2 tbsp. Nutritional Yeast
Dressing Ingredients
1 tbsp. Mayonnaise (no soybean oil) 1 tbsp. White Wine Vinegar
1   tsp. Sour cream 2 tbsp. olive oil
1/2 tsp. Greek seasoning Sea salt

Combine all of the dressing ingredients Combine all of the base salad
ingredients Cut the bacon into squares.
Cook the bacon until brown and crisp over medium high heat.
Crumble them on top of the salad ingredients
Drizzle with vinaigrette

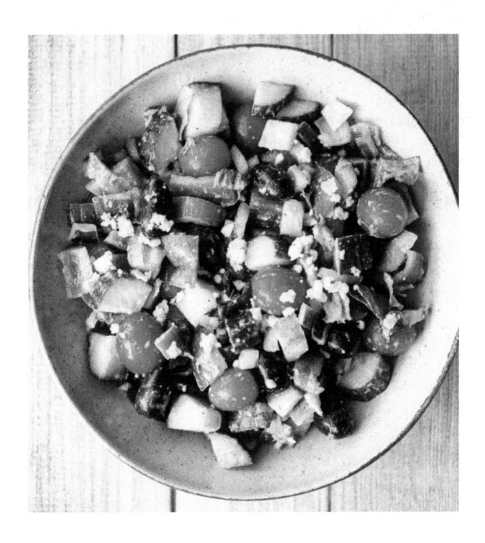

Boston Lettuce with Pistachio Nuts and Bacon Salad

Base Salad Ingredients
2 ¼ oz Boston Lettuce 1/4 cup pistachio nuts
2 slices of bacon
2 tbsp. Nutritional Yeast
Dressing Ingredients
1 tbsp. Mayonnaise (no soybean oil) 1 tbsp. Red Wine Vinegar
1 tsp. Sour cream
2 tbsp. Extra virgin olive oil 1/2 tsp. Herbs de Provence Sea salt

Combine all of the dressing ingredients Combine all of the base salad
ingredients Cut the bacon into squares.
Cook the bacon until brown and crisp over medium high heat.
Crumble them on top of the salad ingredients
Drizzle with vinaigrette

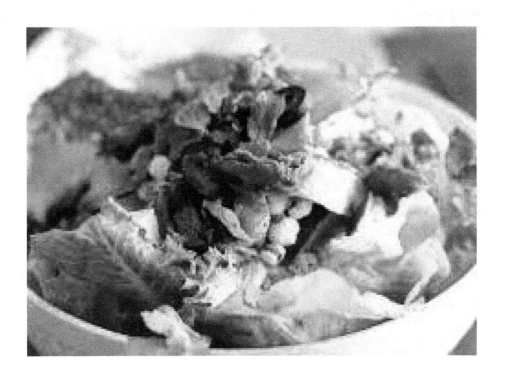

Spicy Broccoli Soup

Ingredients
1 ½ cups vegetable broth
½ cube pork bouillon cube 1 tbsp. Sesame oil
2 large eggs
1 tsp. Chili garlic paste Pinch of Sea salt
½ cup broccoli

Over medium-high heat, vegetable broth, pork bouillon cube and sesame oil. Bring to a boil and add the chili garlic paste.
Turn off the stove.
Beat the eggs lightly. You should still see streaks of white and yellow.
Add to the soup and stir.
Add the vegetables. Season with sea salt.

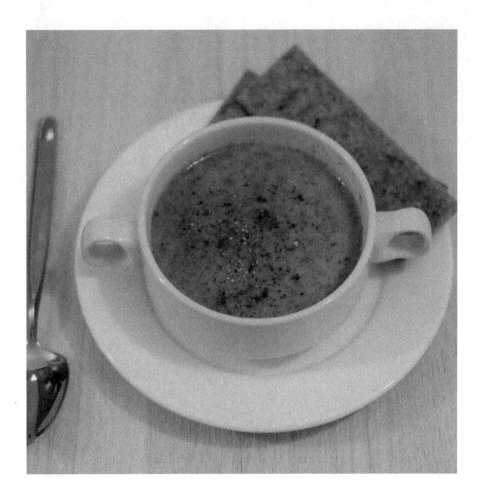

Spicy Cauliflower Soup

Ingredients
1 ½ cups vegetable broth
½ cube pork bouillon cube 1 tbsp. Sesame oil
2 large eggs
1 tsp. Chili garlic paste Pinch of Sea salt
½ cup cauliflower

Over medium-high heat, vegetable broth, pork bouillon cube and sesame oil. Bring to a boil and add the chili garlic paste.
Turn off the stove.
Beat the eggs lightly. You should still see streaks of white and yellow.
Add to the soup and stir.
Add the vegetables. Season with sea salt.

Ù

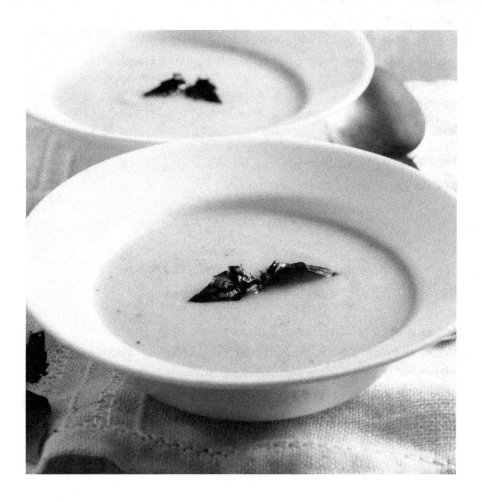

Chicken and Turkey Meatballs

Main Ingredients
½ pound ground chicken
½ pound ground turkey
2   medium yellow onions, chopped
½ medium yellow bell pepper 2 tbsp. Cilantro, finely chopped
½ tsp. cumin
½ tsp. chili powder
½ tsp. Sea Salt
½ tsp. Red pepper flakes
Juice and zest of ¼ medium lemon 2 ounces cashew cheese
2 tbsp. Flaxseed meal 2 tbsp. Almond flour

Guacamole
1 medium avocado
Juice of ⅓ of medium lime 1 tbsp. finely minced garlic Sea Salt
Extra virgin olive oil

Preheat the oven to 350 degrees F.
Combine all of the main ingredients together. Roll them into meatballs
and bake for 18 min. Combine all of the guacamole ingredients.
Serve the meatballs with guacamole.

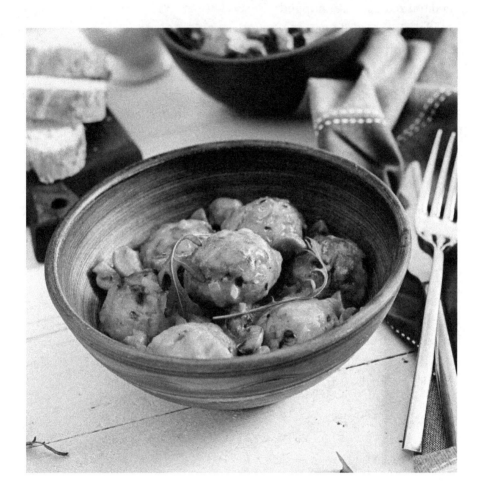

Pork and Beef Meatballs

Main Ingredients
½ pound ground beef
½ pound ground pork
2 medium red onions, chopped
½ medium green bell pepper
2 tbsp. Cilantro, finely chopped
½ tsp. cumin
½ tsp. chili powder
½ tsp. Sea Salt
½ tsp. cayenne pepper
Juice and zest of ¼ medium lime 2 ounces cashew cheese
2 tbsp. Flaxseed meal 2 tbsp. Almond flour

Guacamole
1 medium avocado
Juice of ⅓ of medium lime 1 tbsp. finely minced garlic Sea Salt
Extra virgin olive oil

Preheat the oven to 350 degrees F.
Combine all of the main ingredients together. Roll them into meatballs
and bake for 18 min. Combine all of the guacamole ingredients.
Serve the meatballs with guacamole.

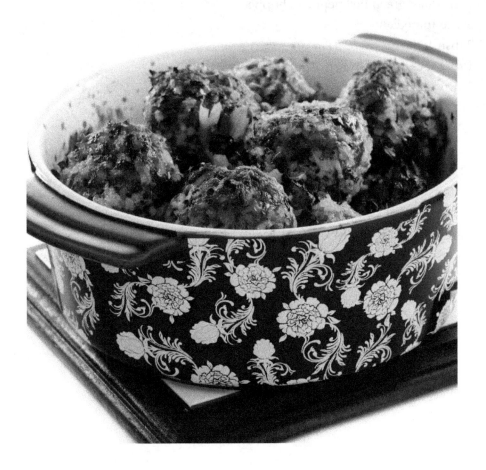

Romaine Lettuce Green Bell Pepper and Sesame Vinaigrette

Salad Ingredients

4 Slices of bacon, cut into squares 2 cups romaine lettuce

¼ cup cilantro, chopped finely

¼ medium green bell pepper, chopped

Sauce Ingredients

2 tbsp. Tomato paste 3 tsp. sea salt

1 tbsp. Sesame oil 3 tbsp. Mayonnaise

½ tsp. sesame seeds

¼ tsp. assorted rainbow peppercorns 4 tsp. apple cider vinegar

½ tsp. Red pepper flakes 2 tbsp. raw honey

Over medium heat, fry the bacon until brown and crisp over medium heat. Combine the salad ingredients.

Combine all of the sauce ingredients.

Toss the salad with the sauce ingredients and top with the bacon

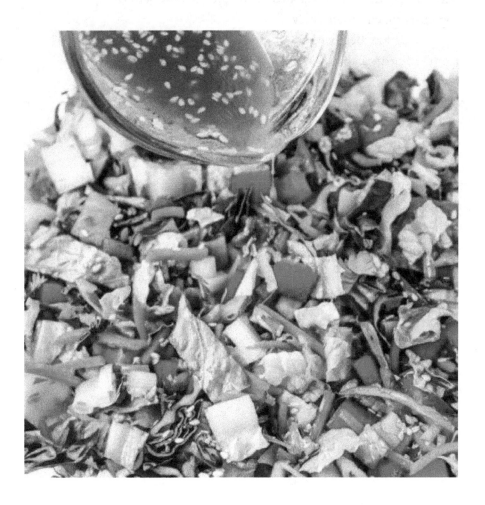

Butter head Lettuce with Cilantro and Bacon Salad

Salad Ingredients

4 Slices of bacon, cut into squares 2 cups butter head lettuce

¼ cup cilantro, chopped finely

¼ medium yellow bell pepper, chopped

Sauce Ingredients 2 tbsp. Tomato paste 3 tsp. sea salt

1 tbsp. extra virgin olive oil 1 tbsp. Tomato sauce

2 tbsp. Chopped parsley Juice & zest of ½ lemon

¼ tsp. Sichuan peppercorns 4 tsp. white wine vinegar

½ tsp. cayenne pepper 2 tbsp. maple syrup

Over medium heat, fry the bacon until brown and crisp over medium heat. Combine the salad ingredients.

Combine all of the sauce ingredients.

Toss the salad with the sauce ingredients and top with the bacon

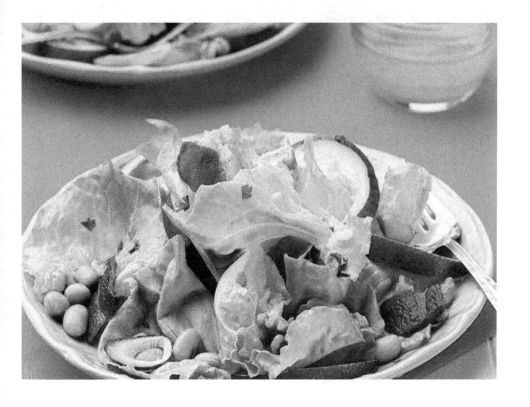

Salmon Onion and Egg Stuffed Avocado Salad

Ingredients

1/2 cup canned salmon

6 large hard-boiled eggs, chopped

⅓ medium yellow onion, chopped 1/2 cup cubed mangoes

¼ cup mayonnaise 2 tsp. mustard

2 tbsp. Fresh lime juice

1 tsp. Frank's red hot sauce

½ tsp. chili powder Sea Salt

3 medium avocados

Boil the seafood until the meat is no longer translucent Combine all of the ingredients in a bowl except the avocado. Slice the avocado and take the seeds out.

Spoon the salad mixture on the avocado.

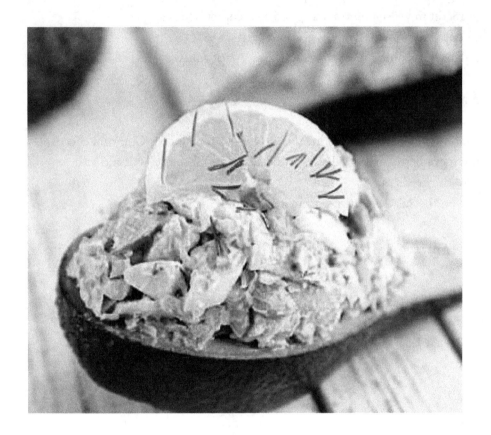

Spicy Shrimp Egg and Onion Stuffed Avocado Salad

Ingredients
6 large shrimps, peeled.
6 large hard-boiled eggs, chopped
⅓ medium yellow onion, chopped 1/2 cup cubed mangoes
¼ cup mayonnaise 2 tsp. Dijon mustard
2 tbsp. Fresh lemon juice 1 tsp. Tabasco hot sauce
½ tsp. Cumin Sea Salt
3 medium avocados

Boil the seafood until the meat is no longer translucent Combine all of the ingredients in a bowl except the avocado. Slice the avocado and take the seeds out.
Spoon the salad mixture on the avocado.

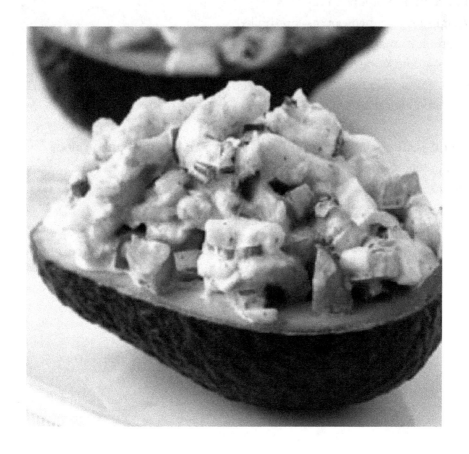

Clams and Egg-Stuffed Avocado Salad with Cashew Cheese

Ingredients

8 large manila clams, shells removed 6 large hard-boiled eggs, chopped
⅓ medium red onion, chopped
1/2 cup finely cubed carrots, pre-boiled
¼ cup mayonnaise 2 tsp. mustard
1 tbsp. White Wine Vinegar 1 tsp. Cashew Cheese
½ tsp. Cumin Sea Salt
3 medium avocados

Boil the seafood until the meat is no longer translucent Combine all of
the ingredients in a bowl except the avocado. Slice the avocado and
take the seeds out.
Spoon the salad mixture on the avocado.

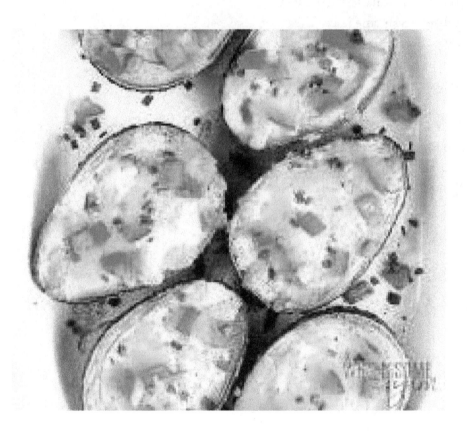

Tuna and Onion-Stuffed Avocado Salad with Spicy Lime Dressing

Ingredients

1/2 cup canned tuna

6 large hard-boiled eggs, chopped

⅓ medium yellow onion, chopped 1/2 cup cubed potatoes, pre-boiled

¼ cup mayonnaise 2 tsp. mustard

2 tbsp. Fresh lime juice

1 tsp. Frank's red hot sauce

½ tsp. chili powder Sea Salt

3 medium avocados

Boil the seafood until the meat is no longer translucent Combine all of the ingredients in a bowl except the avocado. Slice the avocado and take the seeds out.

Spoon the salad mixture on the avocado.

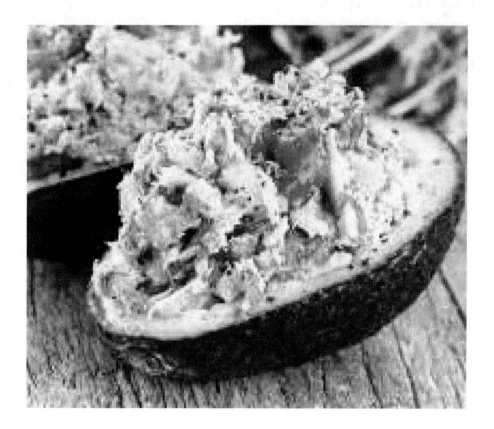

Chicken Bacon and Sun-dried Tomato Pesto Patty

Ingredients

12 ounces chicken thigh, deboned and chopped 4 slices bacon

2 medium yellow bell peppers

¼ cup sun-dried tomato pesto

¼ cup nutritional yeast 1 large egg

3 tbsp. sesame seeds Pinch of sea salt

Fry the bacon until brown and crisp on medium-high heat.

In a food processor, chop the bell peppers and take out the moisture with the paper towel. Put the meat and bacon in the food processor and blend until smooth.

Add and combine this with the rest of the ingredients thoroughly.

Form into patties and fry in medium heat until golden brown.

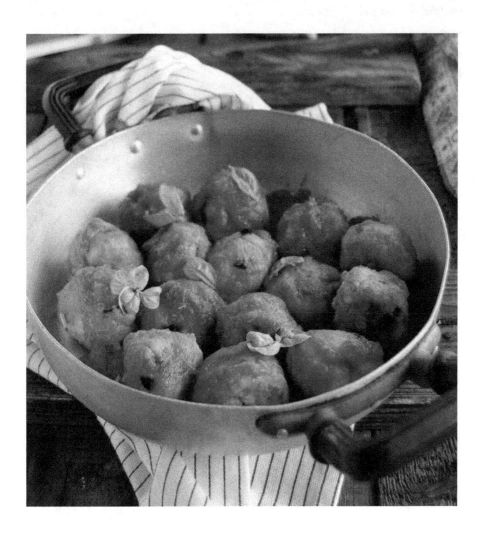

Turkey Bacon and Green Bell Pepper Patty

Ingredients

12 ounces turkey breast, deboned and chopped 4 slices bacon

2 medium green bell peppers

¼ cup salsa

¼ cup cashew cheese 1 large egg

3 tbsp. Almond flour Pinch of sea salt

Fry the bacon until brown and crisp on medium-high heat.

In a food processor, chop the bell peppers and take out the moisture with the paper towel. Put the meat and bacon in the food processor and blend until smooth.

Add and combine this with the rest of the ingredients thoroughly.

Form into patties and fry in medium heat until golden brown.

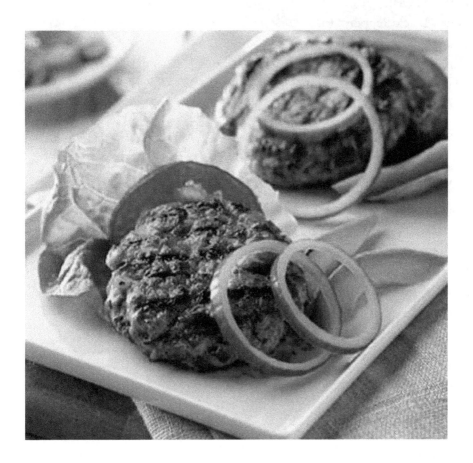

Lamb and Pork Burger in Portobello Bread

Ingredients

1 tbsp. Extra virgin olive oil 1 clove garlic, minced

1 tsp. Greek seasoning

¼ tsp. Sea salt

¼ tsp. Black Peppercorns

2 caps Portobello mushroom caps

Burger Patty

4 ounces ground lamb 2 ounces ground pork 1 egg

1 tsp. Italian seasoning 1 tsp. Sea salt.

¼ cup cashew cheese

Combine oil, salt and spices

Clean the mushrooms by taking out the gills. Marinate them with the oil and the spices

To make the patty, combine all of the burger patty ingredients. Form them into a round patty.

Place the Portobello mushrooms on the grill and cook for 8 min. Add the burger to the grill and cook for 5 min. on each side.

Top with cashew cheese.

Assemble the burger by placing it in between the Portobello mushrooms.

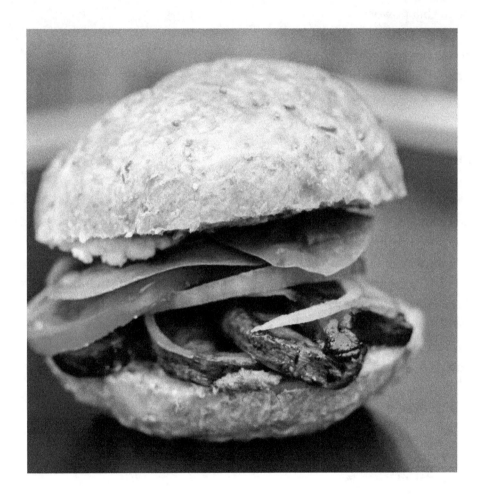

Turkey and Chicken Burger in Portobello Bread with Cashew Cheese

Ingredients

1 tbsp. Extra virgin olive oil 1 clove garlic, minced

1 tsp. chili powder

¼ tsp. Sea salt

¼ tsp. cumin

2 caps Portobello mushroom caps

Burger Patty

5 ounces ground turkey

3 ounces ground chicken thighs 1 egg

1 tsp. Sea salt.

¼ cup cashew cheese

Combine oil, salt and spices

Clean the mushrooms by taking out the gills. Marinate them with the oil and the spices

To make the patty, combine all of the burger patty ingredients. Form them into a round patty.

Place the Portobello mushrooms on the grill and cook for 8 min. Add the burger to the grill and cook for 5 min. on each side.

Top with cashew cheese.

Assemble the burger by placing it in between the Portobello mushrooms.

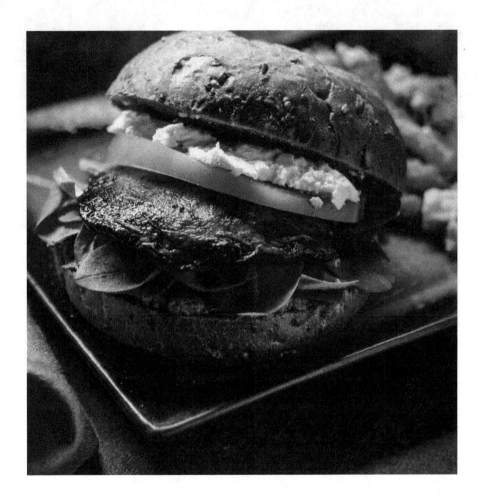

Spicy Roasted Turkey Breast

Ingredients

8 turkey breast Seasoning Ingredients

¾ cup extra virgin olive oil 2 tbsp. chili powder

40 peeled cloves of garlic Sea Salt

Preheat the oven 350 degrees F. Generously season the meat with salt.
In a skillet, pan fry meat with olive oil on medium high heat. Take it
out of the heat and add seasoning ingredients.

Place them in a baking pan and cover. Bake for 1 ½ hours.

Let them rest for 5 to 10 min. Carve and serve.

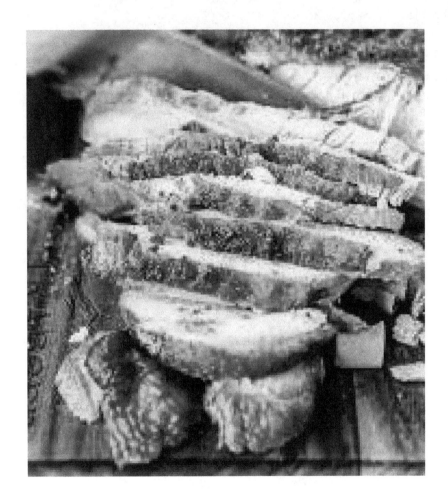

Roasted Pheasant with Thyme

Ingredients
1 Whole Pheasant Quartered Seasoning Ingredients
¾ cup extra virgin olive oil 10 sprigs thyme
40 peeled cloves of garlic Sea Salt

Preheat the oven 350 degrees F. Generously season the meat with salt.
In a skillet, pan fry meat with olive oil on medium high heat. Take it
out of the heat and add seasoning ingredients.
Place them in a baking pan and cover. Bake for 1 ½ hours.
Let them rest for 5 to 10 min. Carve and serve.

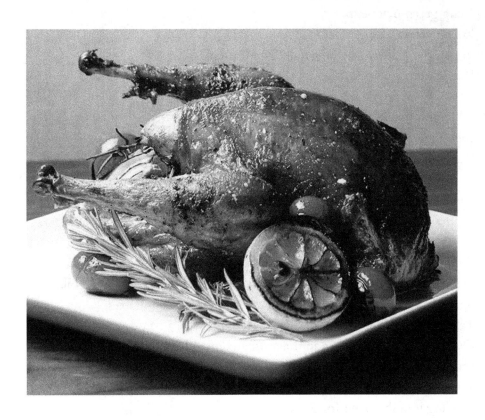

Simple Salmon Cakes

Ingredients
½ pound fresh salmon
¾ cup Olive oil
Sea salt and pepper, to taste Aromatic Ingredients
¾ cup diced red onion 1 cup diced celery
1 cup green bell pepper
½ cup yellow bell pepper
¼ cup flat-leaf parsley, minced 2 tsp. Capers
¼ tsp. Tabasco
½ tsp. Worcestershire sauce 1 ½ tsp.
Old bay seasoning Binding
Ingredients
1 cup almond flour
½ cup mayonnaise
2 tsp. English mustard
2 large eggs, lightly beaten

Preheat the oven to 350 degrees F
Place the fish skin-side down on a sheet pan and brush with olive oil.
Sprinkle some salt and pepper and roast for 15 to 20 minutes.
Take it out of the oven and rest for 10 min.
Over medium low-heat, add the aromatic ingredients Cook until vegetables are tender.
Toast the almond flour by spreading it evenly on a baking sheet and roasting it in the oven for 5 min.
Flake the fish in a large bowl and combine with all of the seasoning and binding ingredients. Chill in the refrigerator for 30 minutes.
Shape them into 10 pcs. of 3-ounce cakes.
Heat the remaining butter and olive oil over medium heat.
Fry the fish cakes for 3 to 4 minutes on each side until browned. Drain and bake in the oven at 250 degrees F.
Rest for 2 min. and serve.

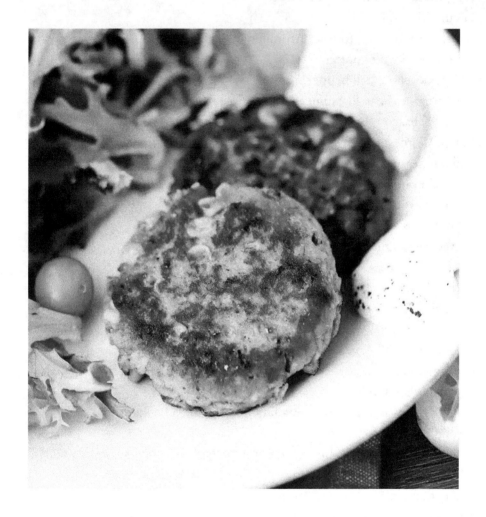

Delicious Halibut Fillet Cakes

Ingredients
1/2 pound Halibut fillets or strips
¾ cup Olive oil
Sea salt and pepper, to taste Aromatic Ingredients
¾ cup diced white onion
1 ½ cups yellow bell pepper
¼ cup flat-leaf parsley, minced 2 tsp. Green Olives
¼ tsp. Tabasco
½ tsp. Worcestershire sauce 1 ½ tsp.
Old bay seasoning Binding Ingredients
1 cup almond flour
½ cup mayonnaise
2 tsp. English mustard
2 large eggs, lightly beaten

Preheat the oven to 350 degrees F
Place the fish skin-side down on a sheet pan and brush with olive oil.
Sprinkle some salt and pepper and roast for 15 to 20 minutes.
Take it out of the oven and rest for 10 min.
Over medium low-heat, add the aromatic ingredients Cook until vegetables are tender.
Toast the almond flour by spreading it evenly on a baking sheet and roasting it in the oven for 5 min.
Flake the fish in a large bowl and combine with all of the seasoning and binding ingredients. Chill in the refrigerator for 30 minutes.
Shape them into 10 pcs. of 3-ounce cakes.
Heat the remaining butter and olive oil over medium heat.
Fry the fish cakes for 3 to 4 minutes on each side until browned. Drain and bake in the oven at 250 degrees F.
Rest for 2 min. and serve.

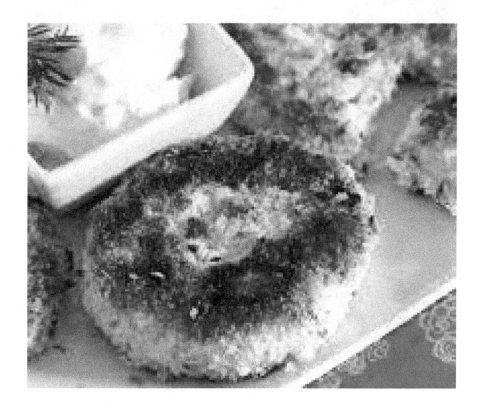

Ground Beef Chuck and Red Onion Meatloaf

Ingredients
1 ¼ lbs. Ground beef chuck 10 tbsp.
cashew cheese Vegetable ingredients
¼ cup chopped red onion
¼ cup chopped green onions
½ cup spinach
¼ cup mushrooms
Seasoning Ingredients
Sea salt and pepper to taste 1 tsp. Garlic powder
½ tsp. paprika
1/2 tsp. marjoram powder

Preheat the oven to 350 degrees F
Combine the meat with the seasoning ingredients.
Grease the loaf pan. Line the bottom and the sides with the meat
mixture. Layer the cheese on the bottom of the meat loaf.
Add the vegetable ingredients
Use the remaining meat to cover the vegetables. Bake for one hour.

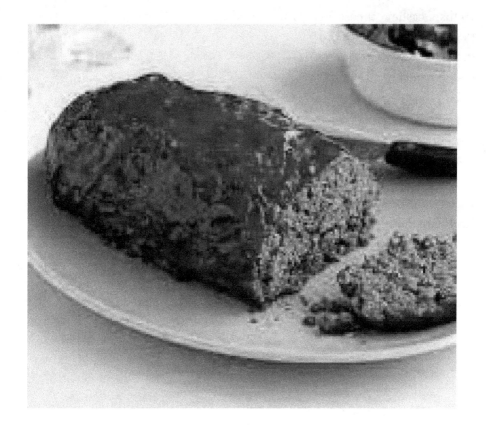

Spicy Ground Chuck Meatloaf

Ingredients

1 lbs. Ground beef chuck

¼ lb. Ground pork

10 tbsp. cashew cheese Vegetable ingredients

¼ cup chopped red onion

¼ cup chopped green onions

½ cup spinach

¼ cup mushrooms

Seasoning Ingredients

Sea salt and pepper to taste 1 tsp. Garlic powder

½ tsp. chili powder

Preheat the oven to 350 degrees F

Combine the meat with the seasoning ingredients.

Grease the loaf pan. Line the bottom and the sides with the meat mixture. Layer the cheese on the bottom of the meat loaf.

Add the vegetable ingredients

Use the remaining meat to cover the vegetables. Bake for one hour.

Jalapeno Broccoli and Beef Chili

Ingredients

4 tbsp. extra virgin olive oil 1 medium red onion, diced 2 lbs. ground chuck

3 ¾ cups chicken broth 3 cups coconut cream 3 tbsp. lemon juice

Aromatic Ingredients

13 ounces canned diced jalapenos 2 tsp. Sea salt

1 tsp. Cumin

½ tsp oregano

1 tsp. Black pepper 1 lb. frozen broccoli

Heat the oil over medium heat in a pressure cooker. Add the onion and meat.

Cook until the onion becomes tender.

Add the aromatic ingredients to the mixture Stir and add 4 cups of broth.

Cover and cook for 30 minutes at high pressure. Let it sit for 10 min. before releasing the steam.

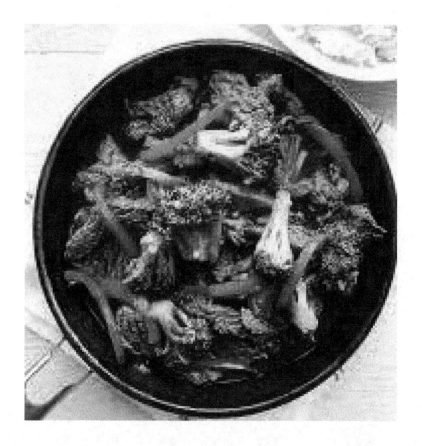

Pork Spinach and Sweet Italian Pepper Chili

Ingredients

4 tbsp. extra virgin olive oil 1 medium red onion, diced 2 lbs. ground pork

3 ¾ cups chicken broth 3 cups coconut cream 3 tbsp. lemon juice

Aromatic Ingredients

11 ounces diced Sweet Italian Peppers 2 tsp. Sea salt

1 tsp. Cumin

½ tsp oregano

1 tsp. Black pepper 1/4 lb. frozen spinach

Heat the oil over medium heat in a pressure cooker. Add the onion and meat.

Cook until the onion becomes tender.

Add the aromatic ingredients to the mixture Stir and add 4 cups of broth.

Cover and cook for 30 minutes at high pressure. Let it sit for 10 min. before releasing the steam.

Fried Herring Fillets

Ingredients

7 ounces Herring fillets or strips 4 tbsp. extra virgin olive oil

2 tbsp. Lemon juice

Dredging Ingredients

¼ cup almond flour 3 tbsp. flax meal

1 tsp. Italian seasoning 1 tsp. Garlic powder

½ tsp. Onion powder Sea Salt to taste

Combine the dredging ingredients thoroughly. Take the fillets and coat them with this mixture.

Heat the oil and add the lemon juice over medium-high heat. Sear the fish for 3 minutes on each side.

Make sure to swirl the pan to keep the fish from sticking. Do not overcook the fish.

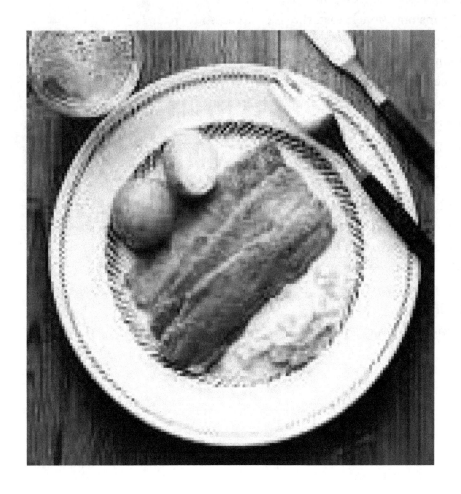

Chicken Thigh and Cauliflower Casserole

Ingredients

1 pound ground boneless chicken thigh 1 small cauliflower, chopped

1 cup cashew cheese, shredded

½ cups nutritional yeast, shredded 1 cup sour cream

Vegetable Ingredients

1 whole jalapeno, chopped

¼ cup chopped green bell pepper

¼ cup chopped red onion Spice Ingredients

1 tsp. Cumin

1 tsp. Cilantro Pinch of turmeric

1 tbsp. Minced garlic

Preheat the oven to 350 degrees F

Place the minced meat and cauliflower in a bowl and add the spice ingredients. Add the vegetable ingredients.

Mix in 1 cup of nutritional yeast Pour this into a casserole dish.

Top with the remaining cashew cheese and nutritional yeast. Bake for 1 hour.

Top with sour cream.

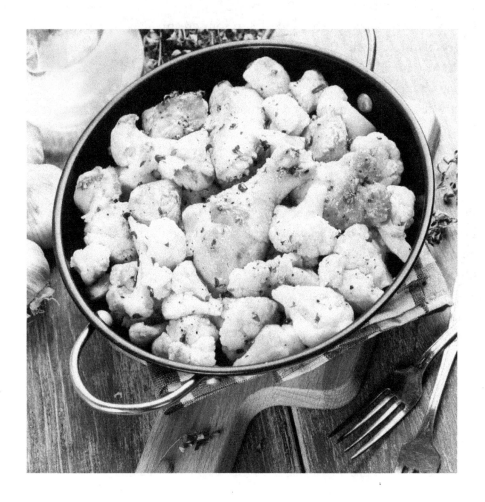

Shrimp Cauliflower and Green Bell Pepper Casserole

Ingredients
1 pound shrimp
1 small cauliflower, chopped
1 cup cashew cheese, shredded
½ cups nutritional yeast, shredded 1 cup sour cream
Vegetable Ingredients
1 whole jalapeno, chopped
¼ cup chopped green bell pepper
¼ cup chopped red onion Spice Ingredients
1 tsp. Cumin
1 tsp. Cilantro Pinch of turmeric
1 tbsp. Minced garlic

Preheat the oven to 350 degrees F
Place the shrimp and cauliflower in a bowl and add the spice ingredients. Add the vegetable ingredients.
Mix in 1 cup of nutritional yeast Pour this into a casserole dish.
Top with the remaining cashew cheese and nutritional yeast. Bake for 1 hour.
Top with sour cream.

Roasted Eggplants

Ingredients

10 medium eggplants, sliced diagonally into chunks

¾ cup extra virgin olive oil 3 tbsp. Italian Seasoning

2 tbsp. Kosher Salt 2 tbsp. raw honey

Preheat the oven to 170 degrees F.

Place the eggplants in a baking pan with the cut side up.

Drizzle with 2/3 cup extra virgin olive oil, raw honey, Italian seasoning and salt. Bake for 10 hours.

Drizzle with the remaining olive oil when you serve.

Cook's Note:

Do this overnight.

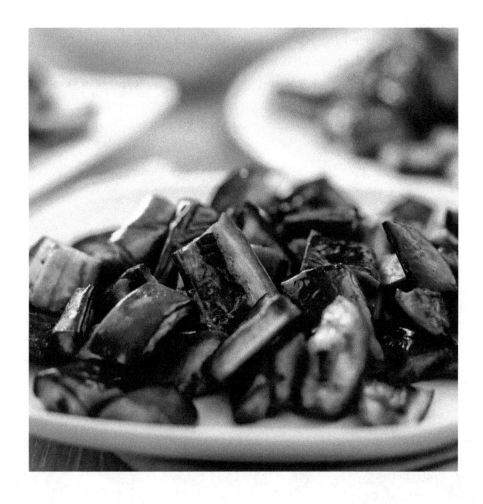

Italian Style Roasted Zucchini

Ingredients

10 medium zucchini, sliced diagonally into chunks

¾ cup extra virgin olive oil 3 tbsp. Italian Seasoning

2 tbsp. Kosher Salt 2 tbsp. raw honey

Preheat the oven to 170 degrees F.

Place the zucchini in a baking pan with the cut side up.

Drizzle with 2/3 cup extra virgin olive oil, raw honey, Italian seasoning and salt. Bake for 10 hours.

Drizzle with the remaining olive oil when you serve.

Cook's Note:

Do this overnight.

Paleo Fried Scallops

Ingredients
2 pounds scallops, shells removed 6 egg whites
2 1/2 cups almond flour Kosher salt

Add the egg whites to the almond flour and mix until smooth.
Dip the seafood into the batter and arrange them on a cookie sheet
Freeze them overnight.
Heat the deep fryer to 375 degrees F. Fry the seafood until pale gold in
color. Season with salt.

Fried Manila Clams

Ingredients

2 pounds manila clams, shells removed 6 egg whites
2 1/2 cups almond flour Kosher salt

Add the egg whites to the almond flour and mix until smooth.
Dip the seafood into the batter and arrange them on a cookie sheet
Freeze them overnight.
Heat the deep fryer to 375 degrees F. Fry the seafood until pale gold in
color. Season with salt.

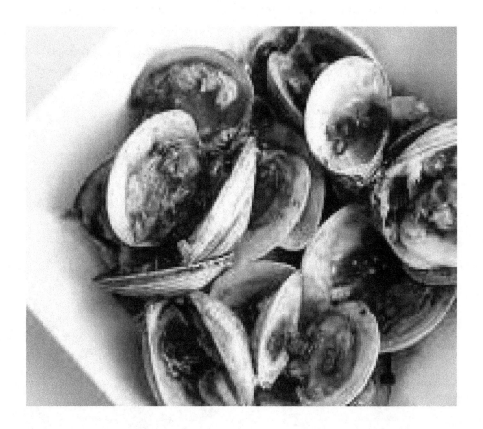

Cod Fillet and Tomato Ceviche

Ingredients

2 pound Cod fillets or strips 4 tomatoes, diced

5 green onions, minced 4 stalks celery, sliced

1 green bell pepper, minced 1 cup chopped fresh parsley freshly
ground black pepper

4 tablespoons extra virgin olive oil

Combine all of the ingredients and chill for one hour.

Herring Fillet Ceviche

Ingredients
2 pound Herring fillets or strips 4 tomatoes, diced
5 green onions, minced 4 stalks celery, sliced
1 green bell pepper, minced 1 cup chopped fresh parsley freshly
ground black pepper
4 tablespoons extra virgin olive oil

Combine all of the ingredients and chill for one hour.

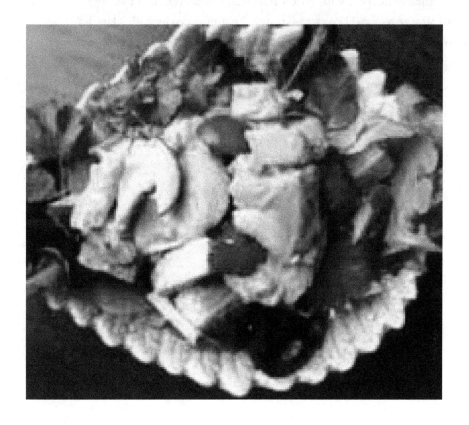

Perfectly Boiled Eggs

Ingredients
3 large eggs
3 pinches of salt

Fill a small saucepan with room temperature water Add the eggs
Bring Water to a boil over maximum heat and cover with glass lid.
Remove the pan from the heat as water starts to bubble.
Keep the lid on.
Take the eggs out of the water after 6

Avocado with Eggs and Cheese

Ingredients

½ medium avocado 3 large eggs

Pinch of kosher salt

1 tbsp. Sliced jalapenos 4 tbsp. Nutritional Yeast 3 tsp. Tajin seasoning

1 tbsp. Extra virgin olive oil Spice Ingredients

1 tsp. Smoked paprika 1 tsp. Onion powder

½ tsp. garlic powder

¼ cup cashew cheese Filling Ingredients

3 ounces chopped cauliflower 3 ounces parsnips, diced

5 ounces eggplant diced

1/2 medium green bell pepper diced

Preheat the oven to 400 degrees F.

Spread all of the filling ingredients and drizzle with olive oil.

Add all of the seasoning ingredients except the cashew cheese and toss to coat. Layer evenly.

Bake for 10 to 15 min. until browned.

Take the vegetables out and top with the cashew cheese. Sliced the avocado in half and take out the seed.

Place the vegetables inside the pit of the avocado.

Add the vegetable mixture and crack the eggs on top of the mixture.

Bake for 10 min.

Top with jalapenos, cashew cheese and tajin.

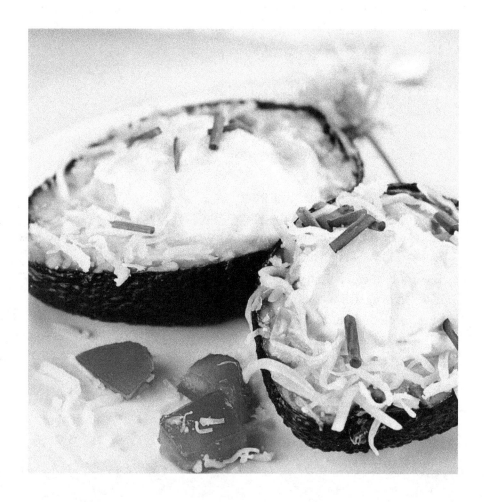

Avocado Stuffed with Zucchini Carrots and Broccoli

Ingredients
½ medium avocado 3 large eggs

Pinch of sea salt

1 tbsp. Sliced jalapenos 4 tbsp. Nutritional Yeast 3 tsp. Tajin seasoning

1 tbsp. Extra virgin olive oil

¼ cup cashew cheese Spice Ingredients

1 tsp. chili powder 1 tsp. Onion powder

½ tsp. garlic powder Filling Ingredients

3 ounces chopped broccoli 3 ounces carrots, diced

5 ounces Zucchini diced

1/2 medium yellow bell pepper diced

Preheat the oven to 400 degrees F.

Spread all of the filling ingredients and drizzle with olive oil.

Add all of the seasoning ingredients except the cashew cheese and toss to coat. Layer evenly.

Bake for 10 to 15 min. until browned.

Take the vegetables out and top with the cashew cheese. Sliced the avocado in half and take out the seed.

Place the vegetables inside the pit of the avocado.

Add the vegetable mixture and crack the eggs on top of the mixture.

Bake for 10 min.

Top with jalapenos, cashew cheese and tajin.

Mexican Grilled Eggplant with Pork Rind

Ingredients

4 tbsp. Olive oil

3 pcs. Chinese egg plant

1 ¼ pounds of ground beef 3 large eggs

1 stalk green onions, thinly sliced 3 cloves garlic crushed

1 small plum tomato diced with seeds removed

¼ tsp. Dried oregano 1 tsp. Ground cumin

½ tsp. Ground coriander 1 tsp. Smoked paprika

½ tsp. onion powder

½ tsp. Chili powder 2 tsp. Sea salt

⅓ cup chopped cilantro 3 tsp. Crushed pork rinds

Broil the eggplant over high heat until the skin becomes tender and browned throughout. In a bowl, beat the egg and set aside.

Heat 1 tbsp. Of olive oil over medium high heat. Add the green onions, garlic and tomato.

Add the oregano, cumin, coriander, paprika, chili powder and salt.

Cook the spices until the consistency resembles a paste.

Add the ground beef. Cook until medium well.

Slit the middle of the eggplant to create a pocket. Flatten and widen the sides.

In another skillet heat the olive oil

Spoon ⅓ of the mixture to the eggplant and pour in the beaten egg to fill up the pocket. Sprinkle with cilantro and place the eggplant on the heated skillet.

Cover with a lid so the eggs can set.

Flip the eggplant until thoroughly cooked. Do the same for the other eggplants.

Sprinkle with pork rinds and cilantro.

Spicy Pan-fried Rib eye with Caramelized Onion

Ingredients
1 tbsp. Extra virgin olive oil
4 pcs. Of 4-ounce ½-inch thick beef rib eye 1 onion cut into strips
1 cup water

Seasoning mixture
½ tsp. Sea salt
½ tsp. Chili Powder
½ tsp. Garlic powder
¼ tsp. Onion powder

Combine all of the ingredients for the seasoning mixture. Rub it all over the meat.
Heat a skillet in medium high heat. Brown the meat while flipping it often. Add the onions and water to the pan.
Reduce the heat and simmer for 20 min.
Turn the meat and cook until water evaporates and onions turn light to medium brown. Remove the meat and top with the onions.

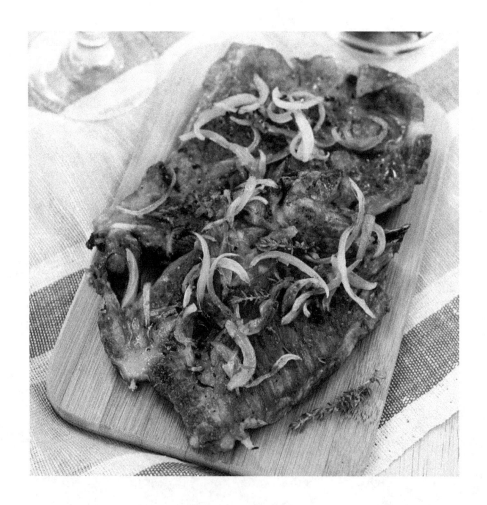

French Style Pan-fried Pork Chop

Ingredients
1 tbsp. Extra virgin olive oil
4 pcs. Of 4-ounce ½-inch thick pork loin chop 1 onion cut into strips
1 cup water

Seasoning mixture
½ tsp. Kosher salt
½ tsp. Herbs de Provence
½ tsp. Garlic powder
¼ tsp. Onion powder

Combine all of the ingredients for the seasoning mixture. Rub it all over the meat.
Heat a skillet in medium high heat. Brown the meat while flipping it often. Add the onions and water to the pan.
Reduce the heat and simmer for 20 min.
Turn the meat and cook until water evaporates and onions turn light to medium brown. Remove the meat and top with the onions.

Smoky roasted Strip loin

Ingredients

4 slices 1-inch thick strip loin

¼ cup extra virgin olive oil 2 tsp. Salt

Spice Ingredients 1 tsp. Cumin

1 tsp. Onion powder

1 tsp. Smoked paprika

Preheat the oven to 400 degrees F

Grease the baking sheet and rub each meat with oil.

Combine the spice ingredients and season all sides of the meat with this mixture.

Place the meat in the baking sheet and bake for 18 min. or until it reaches an internal temperature of 145 degrees F.

Notes: Make sure to take them out at 145 degrees F so you don't lose too much moisture.

Spicy Roasted New York Steak

Ingredients

4 slices 1-inch thick New York Steak

¼ cup extra virgin olive oil 2 tsp. Salt

Spice Ingredients

1 tsp. Garlic powder 1 tsp. Onion powder 1 tsp. Chili powder

Preheat the oven to 400 degrees F

Grease the baking sheet and rub each meat with oil.

Combine the spice ingredients and season all sides of the meat with this mixture.

Place the meat in the baking sheet and bake for 18 min. or until it reaches an internal temperature of 145 degrees F.

Notes: Make sure to take them out at 145 degrees F so you don't lose too much moisture.

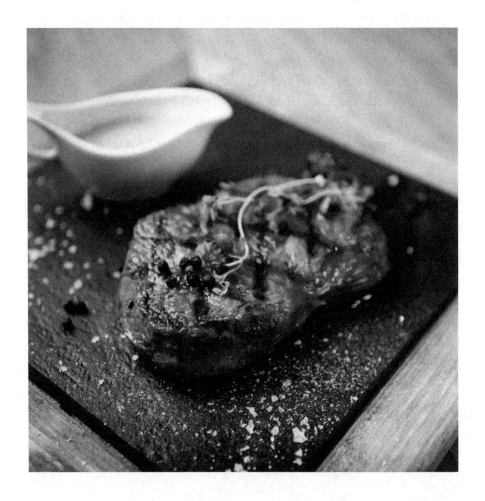

Roasted Striped Bass with Herbs de Provence

Ingredients
4 slices 1-inch thick Striped bass fillets or strips

¼ cup extra virgin olive oil 2 tsp. Salt

Spice Ingredients

1 tsp. Garlic powder 1 tsp. Onion powder

1 tsp. Herbs de Provence

Preheat the oven to 400 degrees F

Grease the baking sheet and rub each fish with oil.

Combine the spice ingredients and season all sides of the fish with this mixture.

Place the fish in the baking sheet and bake for 18 min. or until it reaches an internal temperature of 145 degrees F.

Notes: Make sure to take them out at 145 degrees F so you don't lose too much moisture.

Greek Style Roasted Tuna Fillet

Ingredients

4 slices 1-inch thick Tuna fillets or strips

¼ cup extra virgin olive oil 2 tsp. Salt

Spice Ingredients

1 tsp. Garlic powder 1 tsp. Onion powder

1 tsp. Greek Seasoning

Preheat the oven to 400 degrees F

Grease the baking sheet and rub each fish with oil.

Combine the spice ingredients and season all sides of the fish with this mixture.

Place the fish in the baking sheet and bake for 18 min. or until it reaches an internal temperature of 145 degrees F.

Notes: Make sure to take them out at 145 degrees F so you don't lose too much moisture.

Roasted Rainbow Trout Fillet with Kaffir Lime

Ingredients

4 slices 1-inch thick Rainbow trout fillets or strips

¼ cup Peanut oil 2 tsp. Salt

Spice Ingredients

1 tsp. Garlic powder 1 tsp. Onion powder

1 tsp. finely chopped Kaffir Lime

Preheat the oven to 400 degrees F

Grease the baking sheet and rub each fish with oil.

Combine the spice ingredients and season all sides of the fish with this mixture.

Place the fish in the baking sheet and bake for 18 min. or until it reaches an internal temperature of 145 degrees F.

Notes: Make sure to take them out at 145 degrees F so you don't lose too much moisture.

Baked Striped Bass with Red Onions

Ingredients

4 slices 1-inch thick Striped bass fillets or strips

¼ cup Peanut oil 2 tsp. Salt

Spice Ingredients

1 tsp. Garlic powder 1 tsp. Onion powder

1 tsp. finely chopped red onions

Preheat the oven to 400 degrees F

Grease the baking sheet and rub each fish with oil.

Combine the spice ingredients and season all sides of the fish with this mixture.

Place the fish in the baking sheet and bake for 18 min. or until it reaches an internal temperature of 145 degrees F.

Notes: Make sure to take them out at 145 degrees F so you don't lose too much moisture.

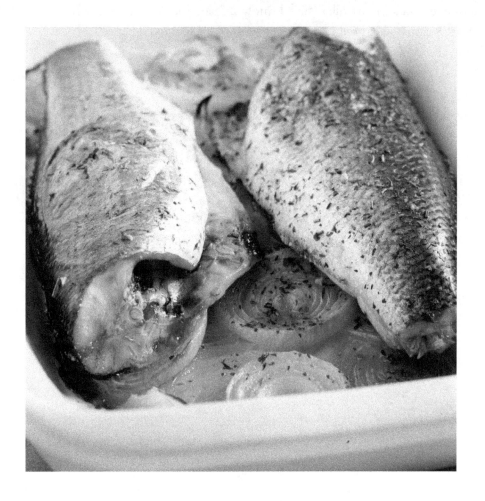

Duck Breast and Cauliflower Stuffed Eggplants

Ingredients
2 large eggplants 4 tbsp. olive oil
3 ounces nutritional yeast, shredded 1 cup cauliflower florets
6 ounces duck breast fillet, sliced thinly 2 tbsp. Sour cream/ dairy free
sour cream 1 stalk green onion
Sea salt, to taste

Preheat the oven to 400 degrees F
Cut the zucchini/eggplant lengthwise and use a melon baller to scoop
out the middle.
Pour 1 tbsp. oil into each zucchini/eggplant and season with salt and
pepper and bake for 20 min. Stir fry the meat on medium high heat.
Stir often until browned.
Cut the florets into small pieces.
Blanch the florets by dipping them into boiling water for 2 min.
Combine the florets and meat with the sour cream.
As the zucchini/eggplant finishes baking, add the meat and vegetable
filling.
Sprinkle the nutritional yeast and bake for 10 to 15 min. or until the
nutritional yeast browns. Garnish with the finely chopped green onion.

Turkey Breast and Green Onion Stuffed Zucchini

Ingredients

2 large zucchini 4 tbsp. olive oil
3 ounces nutritional yeast, shredded 1 cup cauliflower florets
6 ounces turkey breast fillet, sliced thinly 2 tbsp. Sour cream/ dairy free sour cream 1 stalk green onion
Sea salt, to taste

Preheat the oven to 400 degrees F
Cut the zucchini/eggplant lengthwise and use a melon baller to scoop out the middle.
Pour 1 tbsp. oil into each zucchini/eggplant and season with salt and pepper and bake for 20 min. Stir fry the meat on medium high heat. Stir often until browned.
Cut the florets into small pieces.
Blanch the florets by dipping them into boiling water for 2 min.
Combine the florets and meat with the sour cream.
As the zucchini/eggplant finishes baking, add the meat and vegetable filling.
Sprinkle the nutritional yeast and bake for 10 to 15 min. or until the nutritional yeast browns. Garnish with the finely chopped green onion.

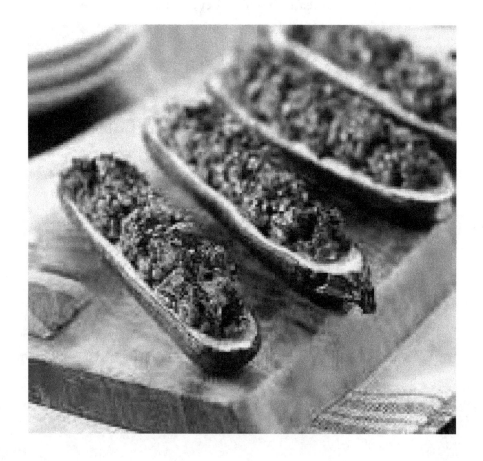

Asian Style Chicken Thigh Stuffed Eggplants

Ingredients

2 large eggplants 4 tbsp. olive oil

3 ounces nutritional yeast, shredded 1 cup broccoli florets

6 ounces chicken thigh fillet, sliced thinly 2 tbsp. Sour cream/ dairy free sour cream 1 stalk green onion

Sea salt, to taste

Preheat the oven to 400 degrees F

Cut the zucchini/eggplant lengthwise and use a melon baller to scoop out the middle.

Pour 1 tbsp. oil into each zucchini/eggplant and season with salt and pepper and bake for 20 min. Stir fry the meat on medium high heat. Stir often until browned.

Cut the florets into small pieces.

Blanch the florets by dipping them into boiling water for 2 min.

Combine the florets and meat with the sour cream.

As the zucchini/eggplant finishes baking, add the meat and vegetable filling.

Sprinkle the nutritional yeast and bake for 10 to 15 min. or until the nutritional yeast browns. Garnish with the finely chopped green onion.

Beef Strip loin Stuffed Zucchini with Sour Cream

Ingredients

2 large zucchini 4 tbsp. olive oil

3 ounces nutritional yeast, shredded 1 cup cauliflower florets

6 ounces beef strip loin, sliced thinly

2 tbsp. Sour cream/ dairy free sour cream 1 stalk green onion

Sea salt, to taste

Preheat the oven to 400 degrees F

Cut the zucchini/eggplant lengthwise and use a melon baller to scoop out the middle.

Pour 1 tbsp. oil into each zucchini/eggplant and season with salt and pepper and bake for 20 min. Stir fry the meat on medium high heat. Stir often until browned.

Cut the florets into small pieces.

Blanch the florets by dipping them into boiling water for 2 min.

Combine the florets and meat with the sour cream.

As the zucchini/eggplant finishes baking, add the meat and vegetable filling.

Sprinkle the nutritional yeast and bake for 10 to 15 min. or until the nutritional yeast browns. Garnish with the finely chopped green onion.

Loose Leaf Lettuce with Cashew Nuts and Bacon Salad

Base Salad Ingredients
2 ¼ oz Loose Leaf Lettuce 1/4 cup cashew nuts
2 slices of bacon
2 tbsp. Nutritional Yeast
Dressing Ingredients
1 tbsp. Mayonnaise (no soybean oil) 1 tbsp. Balsamic Vinegar
1 tsp. Sour cream
2 tbsp. Extra virgin olive oil 1/2 tsp. Greek seasoning Sea salt

Combine all of the dressing ingredients Combine all of the base salad
ingredients Cut the bacon into squares.
Cook the bacon until brown and crisp over medium high heat.
Crumble them on top of the salad ingredients
Drizzle with vinaigrette

Bib Lettuce with Bacon and Macadamia Nut Salad

Base Salad Ingredients
2 ¼ oz Bib Lettuce
1/4 cup macadamia nuts 2 slices of bacon
2 tbsp. Nutritional Yeast
Dressing Ingredients
1 tbsp. Mayonnaise (no soybean oil) 1 tbsp. White Wine Vinegar
1 tsp. Sour cream 2 tbsp. olive oil
1/2 tsp. Herbs de Provence Sea salt

Combine all of the dressing ingredients Combine all of the base salad ingredients Cut the bacon into squares.
Cook the bacon until brown and crisp over medium high heat.
Crumble them on top of the salad ingredients
Drizzle with vinaigrette

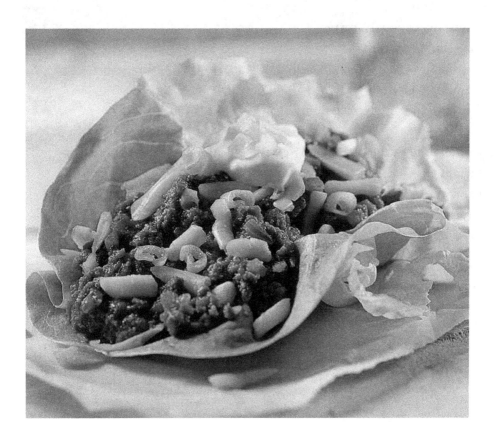

Iceberg Lettuce with Walnuts and Honey Dressing

Base Salad Ingredients
2 ¼ oz Iceberg Lettuce 1/4 cup walnuts
2 slices of bacon
2 tbsp. Nutritional Yeast
Dressing Ingredients
1 tbsp. Mayonnaise (no soybean oil) 1 tbsp. Red Wine Vinegar
1 tsp. Raw Honey
2 tbsp. Extra virgin olive oil 1/2 tsp. Greek seasoning Sea salt

Combine all of the dressing ingredients Combine all of the base salad ingredients Cut the bacon into squares.
Cook the bacon until brown and crisp over medium high heat.
Crumble them on top of the salad ingredients
Drizzle with vinaigrette

Romaine Lettuce with Pine Nuts and Bacon

Base Salad Ingredients
2 ¼ oz Romaine Lettuce 1/4 cup pine nuts
2 slices of bacon
2 tbsp. Nutritional Yeast
Dressing Ingredients
1 tbsp. Mayonnaise (no soybean oil) 1 tbsp. White Wine Vinegar
1 tsp. English Mustard 2 tbsp. olive oil
1/2 tsp. Greek seasoning Sea salt

Combine all of the dressing ingredients Combine all of the base salad
ingredients Cut the bacon into squares.
Cook the bacon until brown and crisp over medium high heat.
Crumble them on top of the salad ingredients
Drizzle with vinaigrette

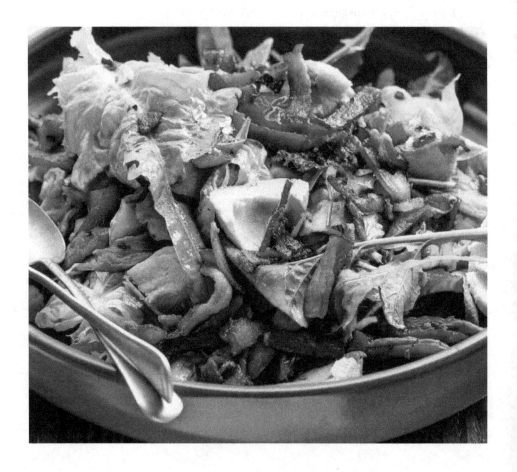

Spicy Wakame Soup

Ingredients
1 ½ cups vegetable broth
½ cube pork bouillon cube 1 tbsp. Sesame oil
2 large eggs
1 tsp. Chili garlic paste Pinch of Sea salt
½ cup Wakame

Over medium-high heat, vegetable broth, pork bouillon cube and sesame oil. Bring to a boil and add the chili garlic paste.
Turn off the stove.
Beat the eggs lightly. You should still see streaks of white and yellow. Add to the soup and stir.
Add the vegetables. Season with sea salt.

Chinese Watercress Soup

Ingredients

1 ½ cups vegetable broth

½ cube pork bouillon cube 1 tbsp. Sesame oil

2 large eggs

1 tsp. Chili garlic paste Pinch of Sea salt

½ cup watercress

Over medium-high heat, vegetable broth, pork bouillon cube and sesame oil. Bring to a boil and add the chili garlic paste.

Turn off the stove.

Beat the eggs lightly. You should still see streaks of white and yellow. Add to the soup and stir.

Add the vegetables. Season with sea salt.

Beef and Lamb Meatballs

Main Ingredients

½ pound ground beef

½ pound ground lamb

2 medium red onions, chopped

½ medium green bell pepper

2 tbsp. Cilantro, finely chopped

½ tsp. cumin

½ tsp. Garlic powder

½ tsp. Sea Salt

½ tsp. Red pepper flakes

Juice and zest of ¼ medium lime 2 ounces cashew cheese

2 tbsp. Flaxseed meal 2 tbsp. Almond flour

Guacamole

1 medium avocado

Juice of ⅓ of medium lime 1 tbsp. finely minced garlic Sea Salt

Extra virgin olive oil

Preheat the oven to 350 degrees F.

Combine all of the main ingredients together. Roll them into meatballs and bake for 18 min. Combine all of the guacamole ingredients. Serve the meatballs with guacamole.

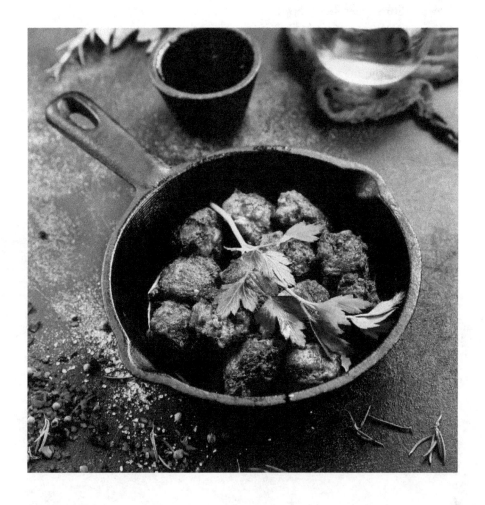

Lamb and Pork Meatballs

Main Ingredients
½ pound ground lamb
½ pound ground pork
1 medium yellow onions, chopped
½ medium green bell pepper
2 tbsp. Cilantro, finely chopped
½ tsp. Onion powder
½ tsp. Cayenne pepper
½ tsp. Sea Salt
½ tsp. Red pepper flakes
Juice and zest of ¼ medium lime 2 ounces cashew cheese
2 tbsp. Flaxseed meal 2 tbsp. Almond flour

Guacamole
1 medium avocado
Juice of ⅓ of medium lime 1 tbsp. finely minced garlic Sea Salt
Extra virgin olive oil

Preheat the oven to 350 degrees F.
Combine all of the main ingredients together. Roll them into meatballs
and bake for 18 min. Combine all of the guacamole ingredients.
Serve the meatballs with guacamole.

Beef Lamb and Yellow Bell Pepper Meatballs

Main Ingredients
½ pound ground beef
½ pound ground lamb
2 medium yellow onions, chopped
½ medium yellow bell pepper 2 tbsp. Cilantro, finely chopped
½ tsp. cumin
½ tsp. chili powder
½ tsp. Sea Salt
½ tsp. Red pepper flakes
Juice and zest of ¼ medium lemon 2 ounces cashew cheese
2 tbsp. Flaxseed meal 2 tbsp. Almond flour

Guacamole
1 medium avocado
Juice of ⅓ of medium lime 1 tbsp. finely minced garlic Sea Salt
Extra virgin olive oil

Preheat the oven to 350 degrees F.
Combine all of the main ingredients together. Roll them into meatballs and bake for 18 min. Combine all of the guacamole ingredients.
Serve the meatballs with guacamole.

Chicken Turkey and Green Bell Pepper Meatballs

Main Ingredients
½ pound ground chicken
½ pound ground turkey
2 medium red onions, chopped
½ medium green bell pepper
2 tbsp. Cilantro, finely chopped
½ tsp. cumin
½ tsp. chili powder
½ tsp. Sea Salt
½ tsp. cayenne pepper
Juice and zest of ¼ medium lime 2 ounces cashew cheese
2 tbsp. Flaxseed meal 2 tbsp. Almond flour

Guacamole
1 medium avocado
Juice of ⅓ of medium lime 1 tbsp. finely minced garlic Sea Salt
Extra virgin olive oil

Preheat the oven to 350 degrees F.
Combine all of the main ingredients together. Roll them into meatballs and bake for 18 min. Combine all of the guacamole ingredients.
Serve the meatballs with guacamole.

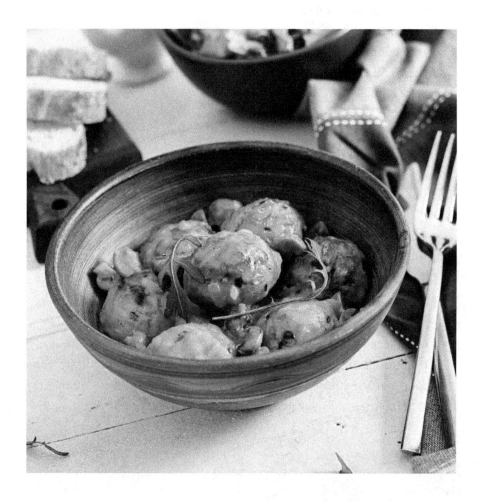

Butter head Lettuce with Yellow Bell Pepper and Tomato Dressing

Salad Ingredients
4 Slices of bacon, cut into squares 2 cups butter head lettuce
¼ cup cilantro, chopped finely
¼ medium yellow bell pepper, chopped
Sauce Ingredients 2 tbsp. Tomato paste 3 tsp. sea salt
1 tbsp. extra virgin olive oil 1 tbsp. Tomato sauce
2 tbsp. Chopped parsley Juice & zest of ½ lemon
¼ tsp. Sichuan peppercorns 4 tsp. white wine vinegar
½ tsp. cayenne pepper 2 tbsp. maple syrup

Over medium heat, fry the bacon until brown and crisp over medium heat. Combine the salad ingredients.
Combine all of the sauce ingredients.
Toss the salad with the sauce ingredients and top with the bacon

Thai Bib Lettuce with Cilantro and Red Curry Dressing

Salad Ingredients
4 Slices of bacon, cut into squares 2 cups bib lettuce

¼ cup cilantro, chopped finely

¼ medium green bell pepper, chopped

Sauce Ingredients 2 tbsp. Tomato paste 3 tbsp. sea salt

1 tbsp. Sesame oil

1 tbsp. Crunchy Peanut Butter 2 tbsp. Chopped cilantro

½ tsp. sesame seeds Juice & zest of ½ lime 1 tsp. Red curry paste

¼ tsp. Sichuan peppercorns 4 tsp. white wine vinegar

½ tsp. Red pepper flakes 1 tsp. Fish sauce

2 tbsp. raw honey

Over medium heat, fry the bacon until brown and crisp over medium heat. Combine the salad ingredients.

Combine all of the sauce ingredients.

Toss the salad with the sauce ingredients and top with the bacon

Broccoli Cauliflower and Turnip Greens Curry

Ingredients
Vegetable Ingredients
½ cup broccoli florets
½ cup cauliflower florets
1 large handful of turnip greens 4 tbsp. Extra virgin coconut oil
¼ medium onion
Aromatic Ingredients 1 tsp. Minced garlic 1 tsp. Minced ginger 3 tsp. Fish sauce
1 tsp. Soy sauce
½ tsp. Sea salt
1 tbsp. Green curry paste 1 tbsp. Sriracha
½ cup coconut milk
Chopped onions and minced garlic

Add 2 tbsp. Coconut oil and cook over medium heat. Add onions and cook until translucent
Add the garlic and cook until golden brown. Turn the heat to medium-low and add the florets.
Keep stirring until the florets are partially cooked. Add the rest of the aromatic ingredients.
Cook for 1 more minute.
Add the remaining vegetable ingredients, coconut cream and coconut oil. Stir together and simmer for 5 to 10 min.

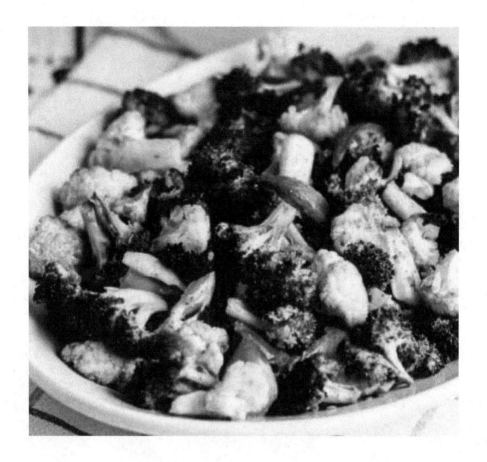

Spicy Cauliflower Curry

Ingredients

Vegetable Ingredients 3/4 cup broccoli florets

1/4 cup cauliflower florets

1 large handful of beet greens 4 tbsp. Extra virgin coconut oil

¼ medium red onion

Aromatic Ingredients 1 tsp. Minced garlic 1 tsp. Minced ginger 3 tsp. Fish sauce

1 tsp. Soy sauce

½ tsp. Sea salt

1 tbsp. red curry paste 1 tbsp. Sriracha

½ cup coconut milk

Chopped onions and minced garlic

Add 2 tbsp. Coconut oil and cook over medium heat. Add onions and cook until translucent

Add the garlic and cook until golden brown. Turn the heat to medium-low and add the florets.

Keep stirring until the florets are partially cooked. Add the rest of the aromatic ingredients.

Cook for 1 more minute.

Add the remaining vegetable ingredients, coconut cream and coconut oil. Stir together and simmer for 5 to 10 min.

Mango and Scallop-Stuffed Avocado Salad

Ingredients

7 large scallops, shells removes

6 large hard-boiled eggs, chopped

⅓ medium yellow onion, chopped 1/2 cup cubed mangoes

¼ cup mayonnaise 2 tsp. Dijon mustard

2 tbsp. Fresh lemon juice

1 tsp. Frank's red hot sauce

½ tsp. Cayenne pepper Sea Salt

3 medium avocados

Boil the seafood until the meat is no longer translucent Combine all of the ingredients in a bowl except the avocado. Slice the avocado and take the seeds out.

Spoon the salad mixture on the avocado.

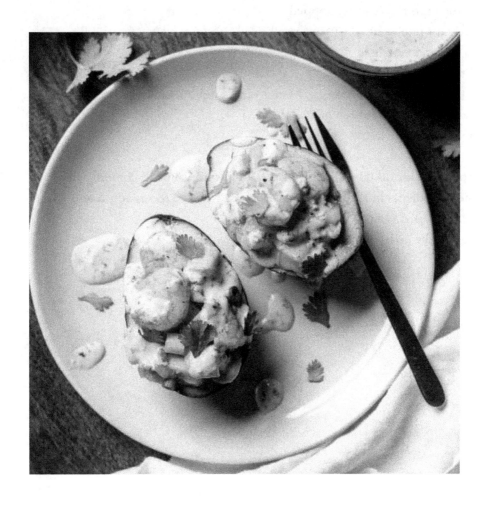

Manila Clam Red Onion and Carrot-Stuffed Avocado Salad

Ingredients

8 large manila clams, shells removed 6 large hard-boiled eggs, chopped
⅓ medium red onion, chopped
1/2 cup finely cubed carrots, pre-boiled
¼ cup mayonnaise
2 tsp. English mustard
1 tbsp. Apple Cider Vinegar 1 tsp. Frank's red hot sauce
½ tsp. chili powder Sea Salt
3 medium avocados

Boil the seafood until the meat is no longer translucent Combine all of the ingredients in a bowl except the avocado. Slice the avocado and take the seeds out.
Spoon the salad mixture on the avocado.

Pork and Yellow Bell Pepper Patty

Ingredients

12 ounces ground pork 4 slices bacon

2 medium yellow bell peppers

¼ cup sun-dried tomato pesto

¼ cup cashew cheese 1 large egg

3 tbsp. Almond flour Pinch of sea salt

Fry the bacon until brown and crisp on medium-high heat.

In a food processor, chop the bell peppers and take out the moisture with the paper towel. Put the meat and bacon in the food processor and blend until smooth.

Add and combine this with the rest of the ingredients thoroughly.

Form into patties and fry in medium heat until golden brown.

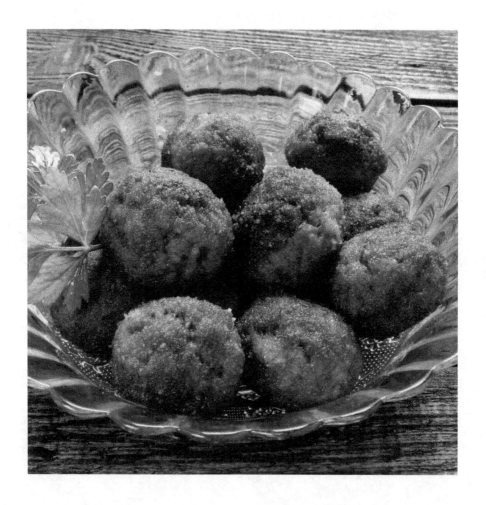

Chuck and Bacon Patty

Ingredients

12 ounces ground chuck 4 slices bacon

2 medium green bell peppers

¼ cup pesto

¼ cup cashew cheese 1 large egg

3 tbsp. Almond flour Pinch of sea salt

Fry the bacon until brown and crisp on medium-high heat.

In a food processor, chop the bell peppers and take out the moisture with the paper towel. Put the meat and bacon in the food processor and blend until smooth.

Add and combine this with the rest of the ingredients thoroughly.

Form into patties and fry in medium heat until golden brown.

Pork and Bacon Patty

Ingredients
12 ounces ground pork 4 slices bacon
2 medium yellow bell peppers
¼ cup tomatillo salsa
¼ cup cashew cheese 1 large egg
3 tbsp. Almond flour Pinch of sea salt

Fry the bacon until brown and crisp on medium-high heat.
In a food processor, chop the bell peppers and take out the moisture
with the paper towel. Put the meat and bacon in the food processor
and blend until smooth.
Add and combine this with the rest of the ingredients thoroughly.
Form into patties and fry in medium heat until golden brown.

Chuck Bacon and Green Bell Pepper Patty

Ingredients
12 ounces ground chuck 4 slices bacon
2 medium green bell peppers
¼ cup sun-dried tomato pesto
¼ cup cashew cheese 1 large egg
3 tbsp. Almond flour Pinch of sea salt

Fry the bacon until brown and crisp on medium-high heat.
In a food processor, chop the bell peppers and take out the moisture with the paper towel. Put the meat and bacon in the food processor and blend until smooth.
Add and combine this with the rest of the ingredients thoroughly.
Form into patties and fry in medium heat until golden brown.

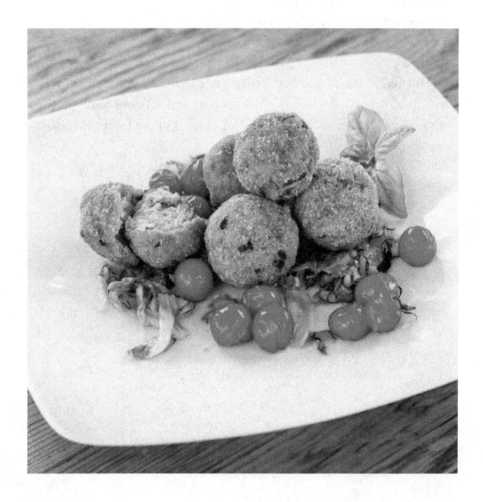

Roast Beef and Jalapeno Lettuce Wraps

Ingredients

5 slices leftover roast beef

½ tsp. sesame seeds 6 pcs. Butter lettuce

2 Jalapeno peppers, sliced into thin strips

¼ Medium Red Onion, sliced into thin strips 2 tsp. Salsa

1 tsp. Extra Virgin Olive oil 1 tsp. Red Pepper Flakes Sea Salt and pepper to taste

Debone the meat.

Shred the meat into small pieces.

Combine the meat with the rest of the ingredients and place them on a piece of butter lettuce. Add some salt and pepper.

Drizzle with sesame seeds Roll the lettuce up.

Beef Brisket Sesame and Lettuce Wraps

Ingredients

10 ounces leftover barbecue beef brisket

½ tsp. sesame seeds 6 pcs. Butter lettuce

⅓ Green Bell Pepper, sliced into thin strips

¼ Medium Red Onion, sliced into thin strips 2 tsp. Garlic Chili Paste

1 tsp. Sesame oil

½ tsp. sesame seeds

½ tsp. Red Pepper Flakes Sea Salt and pepper to taste

Debone the meat.

Shred the meat into small pieces.

Combine the meat with the rest of the ingredients and place them on a piece of butter lettuce. Add some salt and pepper.

Drizzle with sesame seeds Roll the lettuce up.

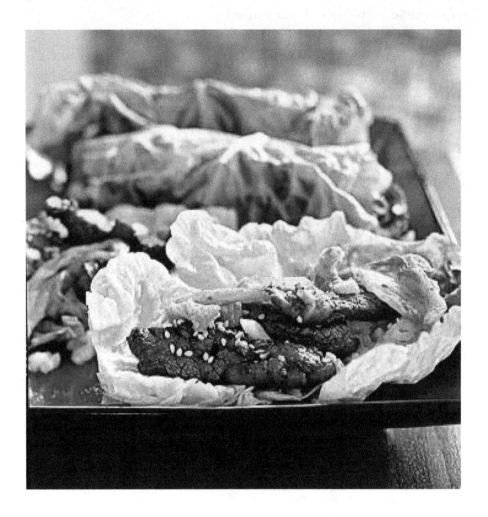

Spicy Lamb Chops with Capers in Lettuce Wraps

Ingredients
3 slices of leftover lamb chops
½ tsp. sesame seeds 6 pcs. Butter lettuce
2 Sweet Italian Peppers, sliced into thin strips
¼ Medium Red Onion, sliced into thin strips 2 tsp. Tabasco Hot Sauce
1 tsp. Olive oil 3/4 tsp. sea salt 1 tsp. capers
1 tsp. kalamata olives
Sea Salt and pepper to taste

Debone the meat.
Shred the meat into small pieces.
Combine the meat with the rest of the ingredients and place them on a piece of butter lettuce. Add some salt and pepper.
Drizzle with sesame seeds Roll the lettuce up.

Pork Shoulder Roast and Jalapeno in Lettuce Wraps

Ingredients

half a pound leftover pork shoulder roast

½ tsp. sesame seeds 6 pcs. Butter lettuce

2 Jalapeno peppers, sliced into thin strips

¼ Medium Red Onion, sliced into thin strips 2 tsp. Salsa

1 tsp. Extra Virgin Olive oil 1 tsp. Red Pepper Flakes Sea Salt and pepper to taste

Debone the meat.

Shred the meat into small pieces.

Combine the meat with the rest of the ingredients and place them on a piece of butter lettuce. Add some salt and pepper.

Drizzle with sesame seeds Roll the lettuce up.

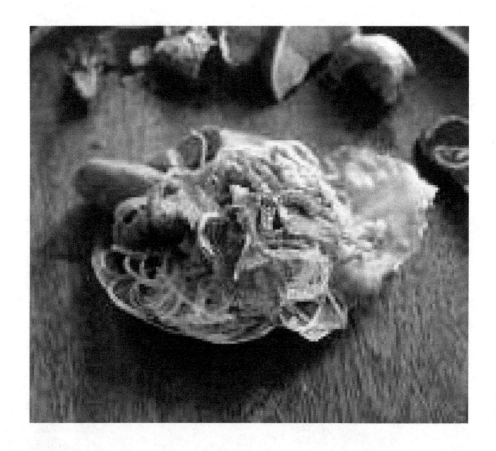

Chuck Burger in Portobello Bread

Ingredients

1 tbsp. Extra virgin olive oil 1 clove garlic, minced

1 tsp. chili powder

¼ tsp. Sea salt

¼ tsp. cumin

2 caps Portobello mushroom caps

Burger Patty

6 ounces ground beef chuck 1 tbsp. English mustard

1 egg

1 tsp. Sea salt.

¼ cup cashew cheese

Combine oil, salt and spices

Clean the mushrooms by taking out the gills. Marinate them with the oil and the spices

To make the patty, combine all of the burger patty ingredients. Form them into a round patty.

Place the Portobello mushrooms on the grill and cook for 8 min. Add the burger to the grill and cook for 5 min. on each side.

Top with cashew cheese.

Assemble the burger by placing it in between the Portobello mushrooms.

Sirloin and Pork Burger in Portobello Burger

Ingredients

1 tbsp. olive oil

1 clove garlic, minced 1 tsp. Greek seasoning

¼ tsp. Sea salt

¼ tsp. Rainbow Peppercorns

2 caps Portobello mushroom caps

Burger Patty

3 ounces ground beef sirloin 3 ounces ground pork

1 tbsp. Dijon mustard 1 tsp. Sea salt.

¼ cup cashew cheese

Combine oil, salt and spices

Clean the mushrooms by taking out the gills. Marinate them with the oil and the spices

To make the patty, combine all of the burger patty ingredients. Form them into a round patty.

Place the Portobello mushrooms on the grill and cook for 8 min. Add the burger to the grill and cook for 5 min. on each side.

Top with cashew cheese.

Assemble the burger by placing it in between the Portobello mushrooms.

Chicken Burger in Portobello Bread

Ingredients
1 tbsp. Extra virgin olive oil 1 clove garlic, minced
1 tsp. Greek seasoning
¼ tsp. Sea salt
¼ tsp. Black Peppercorns
2 caps Portobello mushroom caps
Burger Patty
6 ounces ground chicken thighs 1 egg
1 tsp. Sea salt.
¼ cup cashew cheese

Combine oil, salt and spices
Clean the mushrooms by taking out the gills. Marinate them with the oil and the spices
To make the patty, combine all of the burger patty ingredients. Form them into a round patty.
Place the Portobello mushrooms on the grill and cook for 8 min. Add the burger to the grill and cook for 5 min. on each side.
Top with cashew cheese.
Assemble the burger by placing it in between the Portobello mushrooms.

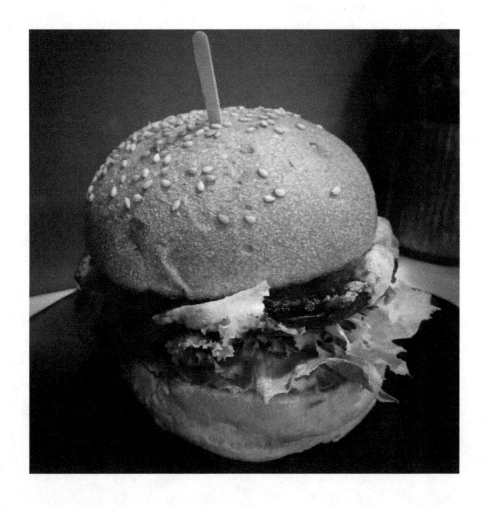

Pork Burger in Portobello Bread

Ingredients
1 tbsp. Extra virgin olive oil 1 clove garlic, minced
1 tsp. chili powder
¼ tsp. Sea salt
¼ tsp. cumin
2 caps Portobello mushroom caps
Burger Patty
6 ounces ground pork 1 tbsp. raw honey
1 tbsp. chili powder 1/2 tsp. cayenne pepper 1 tsp. Sea salt.
¼ cup cashew cheese

Combine oil, salt and spices
Clean the mushrooms by taking out the gills. Marinate them with the oil and the spices
To make the patty, combine all of the burger patty ingredients. Form them into a round patty.
Place the Portobello mushrooms on the grill and cook for 8 min. Add the burger to the grill and cook for 5 min. on each side.
Top with cashew cheese.
Assemble the burger by placing it in between the Portobello mushrooms.

Crispy Pan-fried Herring Fillet

Ingredients Dredging Ingredients Sea salt, to taste
Flax meal for dredging Main Ingredients
1 large Herring fillet 2 tbsp. Olive oil
3 tbsp. Butter Garnishing Ingredients 1 tbsp. Capers, drained Juice of 1 lemon

Season the fish with salt
Coat the fish with the remaining dredging ingredients. Heat the butter with the olive oil.
As soon as it starts to foam, place fish skin-side down. Jiggle the pan to keep the skin from sticking. Cook until a crust forms. Flip the fish and jiggle for a few seconds once more to keep it from sticking.
Cook until golden brown.
Fry the garnishing ingredients except the juice with the remaining fat
Sprinkle with juice once it's finished.
Pour the sauce over the fish.

Pan-fried Mahi-mahi Fillet

Ingredients Dredging Ingredients Sea salt, to taste
Crushed Pork Rinds for dredging Main Ingredients
1 large Mahi-mahi fillet 2 tbsp. Olive oil
3 tbsp. Butter Garnishing Ingredients 1 tbsp. Capers, drained Juice of 1
lemon

Season the fish with salt
Coat the fish with the remaining dredging ingredients. Heat the butter
with the olive oil.
As soon as it starts to foam, place fish skin-side down. Jiggle the pan to
keep the skin from sticking. Cook until a crust forms. Flip the fish and
jiggle for a few seconds once more to keep it from sticking.
Cook until golden brown.
Fry the garnishing ingredients except the juice with the remaining fat
Sprinkle with juice once it's finished.
Pour the sauce over the fish.

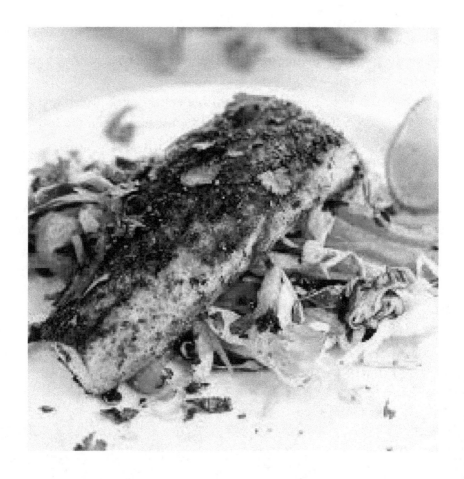

Pan-fried Pollock Fillet

Ingredients Dredging Ingredients Sea salt, to taste
Coconut Flour for dredging Main Ingredients
1 large Pollock fillet 2 tbsp. Olive oil
3 tbsp. Butter Garnishing Ingredients 1 tbsp. Capers, drained Juice of 1
lemon

Season the fish with salt
Coat the fish with the remaining dredging ingredients. Heat the butter
with the olive oil.
As soon as it starts to foam, place fish skin-side down. Jiggle the pan to
keep the skin from sticking. Cook until a crust forms. Flip the fish and
jiggle for a few seconds once more to keep it from sticking.
Cook until golden brown.
Fry the garnishing ingredients except the juice with the remaining fat
Sprinkle with juice once it's finished.
Pour the sauce over the fish.

Spicy Pan-fried Lemon sole Fillet

Ingredients Dredging Ingredients Sea salt, to taste
1 cup Almond flour for dredging 1/2 tsp. Cayenne Pepper
Main Ingredients
1 large Lemon sole fillet 2 tbsp. Olive oil
3 tbsp. Butter Garnishing Ingredients 1 tbsp. Capers, drained Juice of 1
lemon

Season the fish with salt
Coat the fish with the remaining dredging ingredients. Heat the butter
with the olive oil.
As soon as it starts to foam, place fish skin-side down. Jiggle the pan to
keep the skin from sticking. Cook until a crust forms. Flip the fish and
jiggle for a few seconds once more to keep it from sticking.
Cook until golden brown.
Fry the garnishing ingredients except the juice with the remaining fat
Sprinkle with juice once it's finished.
Pour the sauce over the fish.

Roasted Garlic Chicken Thighs

Ingredients

8 chicken thighs Seasoning Ingredients

¾ cup extra virgin olive oil 10 sprigs thyme

40 peeled cloves of garlic Sea Salt

Preheat the oven 350 degrees F. Generously season the meat with salt. In a skillet, pan fry meat with olive oil on medium high heat. Take it out of the heat and add seasoning ingredients.

Place them in a baking pan and cover. Bake for 1 ½ hours.

Let them rest for 5 to 10 min. Carve and serve.

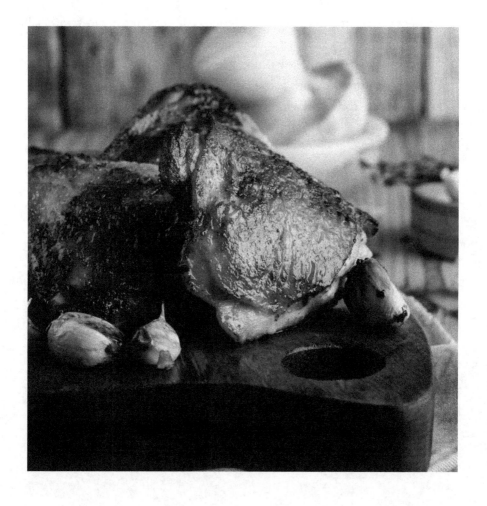

Roasted Chili Garlic Turkey Drumsticks

Ingredients
8 turkey drumsticks Seasoning Ingredients
¾ cup sesame oil Chili Garlic Sauce
20 peeled cloves of garlic Sea Salt

Preheat the oven 350 degrees F. Generously season the meat with salt.
In a skillet, pan fry meat with olive oil on medium high heat. Take it
out of the heat and add seasoning ingredients.
Place them in a baking pan and cover. Bake for 1 ½ hours.
Let them rest for 5 to 10 min. Carve and serve.

Delicious Herring Fillet Cakes with Yellow Bell Pepper

Ingredients
1/2 pound Herring fillets or strips
¾ cup Olive oil
Sea salt and pepper, to taste Aromatic Ingredients
¾ cup diced white onion
1 ½ cups yellow bell pepper
¼ cup flat-leaf parsley, minced 2 tsp. Green Olives
¼ tsp. Tabasco
½ tsp. Worcestershire sauce 1 ½ tsp. Old bay seasoning Binding

Ingredients
1 cup almond flour
½ cup mayonnaise
2 tsp. English mustard
2 large eggs, lightly beaten

Preheat the oven to 350 degrees F
Place the fish skin-side down on a sheet pan and brush with olive oil.
Sprinkle some salt and pepper and roast for 15 to 20 minutes.
Take it out of the oven and rest for 10 min.
Over medium low-heat, add the aromatic ingredients Cook until vegetables are tender.
Toast the almond flour by spreading it evenly on a baking sheet and roasting it in the oven for 5 min.
Flake the fish in a large bowl and combine with all of the seasoning and binding ingredients. Chill in the refrigerator for 30 minutes.
Shape them into 10 pcs. of 3-ounce cakes.
Heat the remaining butter and olive oil over medium heat.
Fry the fish cakes for 3 to 4 minutes on each side until browned. Drain and bake in the oven at 250 degrees F.
Rest for 2 min. and serve.

Delicious Mahi-mahi Fillet Cakes with Celery and Green Bell Pepper

Ingredients

1/2 pound Mahi-mahi fillets or strips

¾ cup Olive oil

Sea salt and pepper, to taste Aromatic Ingredients

¾ cup diced yellow onion 1 cup diced celery

1 1/2 cups green bell pepper

¼ cup flat-leaf parsley, minced 2 tsp. Capers

¼ tsp. Tabasco

½ tsp. Worcestershire sauce 1 ½ tsp. Old bay seasoning Binding

Ingredients

1 cup almond flour

½ cup mayonnaise

2 tsp. English mustard

2 large eggs, lightly beaten

Preheat the oven to 350 degrees F

Place the fish skin-side down on a sheet pan and brush with olive oil.

Sprinkle some salt and pepper and roast for 15 to 20 minutes.

Take it out of the oven and rest for 10 min.

Over medium low-heat, add the aromatic ingredients Cook until vegetables are tender.

Toast the almond flour by spreading it evenly on a baking sheet and roasting it in the oven for 5 min.

Flake the fish in a large bowl and combine with all of the seasoning and binding ingredients. Chill in the refrigerator for 30 minutes.

Shape them into 10 pcs. of 3-ounce cakes.

Heat the remaining butter and olive oil over medium heat.

Fry the fish cakes for 3 to 4 minutes on each side until browned. Drain and bake in the oven at 250 degrees F.

Rest for 2 min. and serve.

Sole Fillet Cakes and Green Bell Peppers

Ingredients
1/2 pound Sole fillets or strips
¾ cup Olive oil
Sea salt and pepper, to taste Aromatic Ingredients
¾ cup diced yellow onion 1 cup diced celery
1 1/2 cups green bell pepper
¼ cup flat-leaf parsley, minced 2 tsp. Capers
¼ tsp. Tabasco
½ tsp. Worcestershire sauce 1 ½ tsp. Old bay seasoning Binding

Ingredients
1 cup almond flour
½ cup mayonnaise
2 tsp. English mustard
2 large eggs, lightly beaten

Preheat the oven to 350 degrees F
Place the fish skin-side down on a sheet pan and brush with olive oil.
Sprinkle some salt and pepper and roast for 15 to 20 minutes.
Take it out of the oven and rest for 10 min.
Over medium low-heat, add the aromatic ingredients Cook until vegetables are tender.
Toast the almond flour by spreading it evenly on a baking sheet and roasting it in the oven for 5 min.
Flake the fish in a large bowl and combine with all of the seasoning and binding ingredients. Chill in the refrigerator for 30 minutes.
Shape them into 10 pcs. of 3-ounce cakes.
Heat the remaining butter and olive oil over medium heat.
Fry the fish cakes for 3 to 4 minutes on each side until browned. Drain and bake in the oven at 250 degrees F.
Rest for 2 min. and serve.

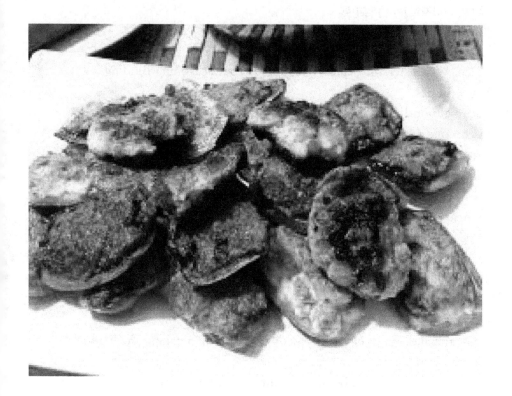

Tilapia Fillet Cakes and Assorted Bell Peppers

Ingredients

1/2 pound Tilapia fillets or strips

¾ cup Olive oil

Sea salt and pepper, to taste Aromatic Ingredients

¾ cup diced red onion 1 cup diced celery

1 cup green bell pepper

½ cup yellow bell pepper

¼ cup flat-leaf parsley, minced 2 tsp. Capers

¼ tsp. Tabasco

½ tsp. Worcestershire sauce 1 ½ tsp. Old bay seasoning Binding

Ingredients

1 cup almond flour

½ cup mayonnaise

2 tsp. English mustard

2 large eggs, lightly beaten

Preheat the oven to 350 degrees F

Place the fish skin-side down on a sheet pan and brush with olive oil.

Sprinkle some salt and pepper and roast for 15 to 20 minutes.

Take it out of the oven and rest for 10 min.

Over medium low-heat, add the aromatic ingredients Cook until vegetables are tender.

Toast the almond flour by spreading it evenly on a baking sheet and roasting it in the oven for 5 min.

Flake the fish in a large bowl and combine with all of the seasoning and binding ingredients. Chill in the refrigerator for 30 minutes.

Shape them into 10 pcs. of 3-ounce cakes.

Heat the remaining butter and olive oil over medium heat.

Fry the fish cakes for 3 to 4 minutes on each side until browned. Drain and bake in the oven at 250 degrees F.

Rest for 2 min. and serve.

Ground Lamb Pork and Beef Meatloaf

Ingredients

¼ lbs. Ground Lamb 1/2 lbs. ground pork 1/2 lbs. ground beef

10 tbsp. cashew cheese Vegetable ingredients

¼ cup chopped red onion

¼ cup chopped green onions

½ cup spinach

¼ cup mushrooms

Seasoning Ingredients

Sea salt and pepper to taste 1 tsp. onion powder

½ tsp. Italian seasoning

Preheat the oven to 350 degrees F

Combine the meat with the seasoning ingredients.

Grease the loaf pan. Line the bottom and the sides with the meat mixture. Layer the cheese on the bottom of the meat loaf.

Add the vegetable ingredients

Use the remaining meat to cover the vegetables. Bake for one hour.

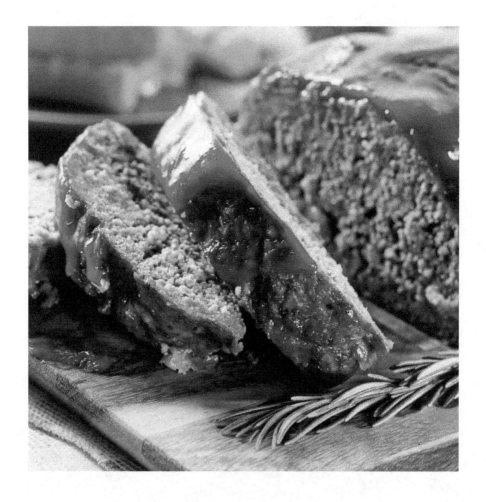

Greek Ground Chuck and Sirloin Meatloaf

Ingredients

¼ lbs. Ground chuck 1/2 lb. ground sirloin 1/2 lb. ground beef

10 tbsp. cashew cheese Vegetable ingredients

¼ cup chopped red onion

¼ cup chopped green onions

½ cup spinach

¼ cup mushrooms

Seasoning Ingredients

Sea salt and pepper to taste 1 tsp. Garlic powder

½ tsp. Greek seasoning

Preheat the oven to 350 degrees F

Combine the meat with the seasoning ingredients.

Grease the loaf pan. Line the bottom and the sides with the meat mixture. Layer the cheese on the bottom of the meat loaf.

Add the vegetable ingredients

Use the remaining meat to cover the vegetables. Bake for one hour.

Onion and Garlic Lamb Pork and Beef Meatloaf

Ingredients

¼ lbs. Ground Lamb 1/2 lbs. ground pork 1/2 lbs. ground beef

10 tbsp. cashew cheese Vegetable ingredients

¼ cup chopped red onion

¼ cup chopped green onions

½ cup spinach

¼ cup mushrooms

Seasoning Ingredients

Sea salt and pepper to taste 1 tsp. Garlic powder

½ tsp. onion powder

Preheat the oven to 350 degrees F

Combine the meat with the seasoning ingredients.

Grease the loaf pan. Line the bottom and the sides with the meat mixture. Layer the cheese on the bottom of the meat loaf.

Add the vegetable ingredients

Use the remaining meat to cover the vegetables. Bake for one hour.

Italian Onion Chuck and Beef Meatloaf

Ingredients

¼ lbs. Ground chuck 1/2 lb. ground sirloin 1/2 lb. ground beef

10 tbsp. cashew cheese Vegetable ingredients

¼ cup chopped red onion

¼ cup chopped green onions

½ cup spinach

¼ cup mushrooms

Seasoning Ingredients

Sea salt and pepper to taste 1 tsp. onion powder

½ tsp. Italian seasoning

Preheat the oven to 350 degrees F

Combine the meat with the seasoning ingredients.

Grease the loaf pan. Line the bottom and the sides with the meat mixture. Layer the cheese on the bottom of the meat loaf.

Add the vegetable ingredients

Use the remaining meat to cover the vegetables. Bake for one hour.

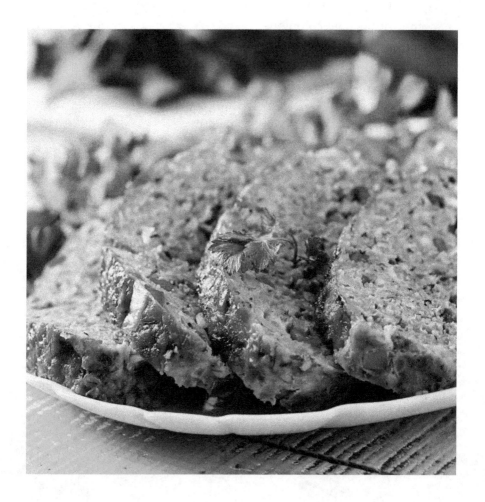

Spanish Roasted Salmon

Ingredients
1 1/4 lb. pound Alaskan salmon fillets or strips Sea salt, to taste
Marinade ingredients
5 tbsp. extra virgin olive oil 3 tbsp. annatto seeds
3 tbsp. apple cider vinegar

Cut the fish into 2 large pieces of fillet. Sprinkle with salt and sit for 30 minutes. Combine the marinade ingredients
Marinate the salmon with this mixture overnight. Preheat the oven to 400 degrees F.
Wipe the marinade off the surface of the fish.
Grease the baking dish and bake the fish for 25 minutes.

Roasted Cod Fillets with Balsamic Sauce

Ingredients
1 1/4 lb. pound Cod fillets or strips Sea salt, to taste
Marinade ingredients
5 tbsp. extra virgin olive oil 1/2 tsp. Italian seasoning
3 tbsp. balsamic vinegar

Cut the fish into 2 large pieces of fillet. Sprinkle with salt and sit for 30 minutes. Combine the marinade ingredients
Marinate the salmon with this mixture overnight. Preheat the oven to 400 degrees F.
Wipe the marinade off the surface of the fish.
Grease the baking dish and bake the fish for 25 minutes.

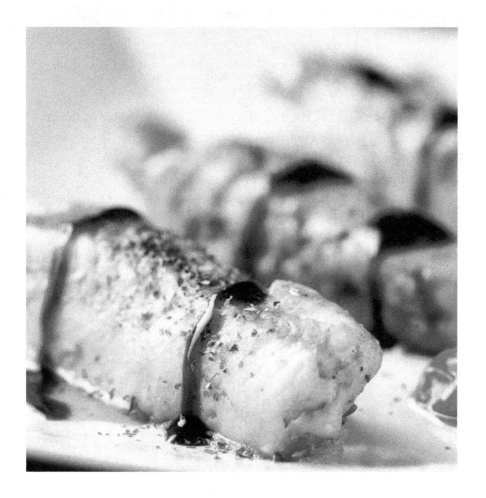

Poached Brussel Sprouts Turnips and Mini Cabbage

Ingredients

1/2 lb. brussel sprouts 1/2 lb. mini cabbage 1/2 lb. turnips, cubed

1/3 cup low sodium vegetable broth

Pinch kosher salt

2 tbsp. extra virgin olive oil 1 tbsp. apple cider vinegar

Place the vegetables on the bottom of a pan and add the water or broth and salt. Cover with lid and cook over high heat for 3 min.

Decrease the heat to low and cook for 3 min.

Remove from the heat and add the rest of the ingredients.

Smoky Pork Casserole

Ingredients

1 pound ground pork

1 small cauliflower, chopped

1 cup cashew cheese, shredded

½ cups nutritional yeast, shredded 1 cup sour cream

Vegetable Ingredients

1 whole jalapeno, chopped

¼ cup chopped green bell pepper

¼ cup chopped red onion Spice Ingredients

1 tsp. Cumin

1 tsp. Cilantro Pinch of turmeric

1 tbsp. Minced garlic

Preheat the oven to 350 degrees F

Place the minced meat and cauliflower in a bowl and add the spice ingredients. Add the vegetable ingredients.

Mix in 1 cup of nutritional yeast Pour this into a casserole dish.

Top with the remaining cashew cheese and nutritional yeast. Bake for 1 hour.

Top with sour cream.

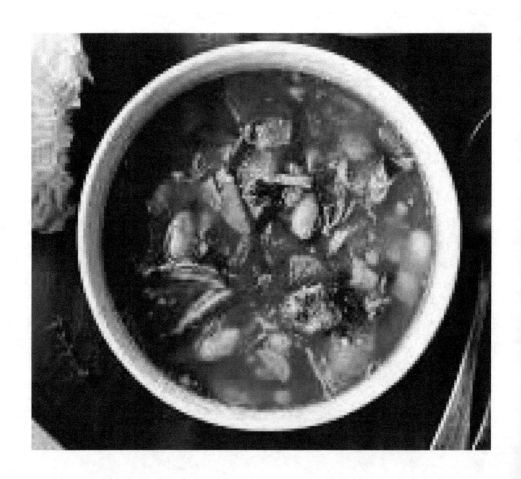

Chicken Bell Pepper and Jalapeno Casserole

Ingredients
1 pound ground chicken
1 small cauliflower, chopped
1 cup cashew cheese, shredded
½ cups nutritional yeast, shredded 1 cup sour cream
Vegetable Ingredients
1 whole jalapeno, chopped
¼ cup chopped green bell pepper
¼ cup chopped red onion Spice Ingredients
1 tsp. Cumin
1 tsp. Cilantro Pinch of turmeric
1 tbsp. Minced garlic

Preheat the oven to 350 degrees F
Place the minced meat and cauliflower in a bowl and add the spice ingredients. Add the vegetable ingredients.
Mix in 1 cup of nutritional yeast Pour this into a casserole dish.
Top with the remaining cashew cheese and nutritional yeast. Bake for 1 hour.
Top with sour cream.

Roasted Purple Yam with Maple Syrup

Ingredients

10 medium purple yam, sliced diagonally into chunks

¾ cup extra virgin olive oil 3 tbsp. Italian Seasoning

2 tbsp. Kosher Salt 2 tbsp. maple syrup

Preheat the oven to 170 degrees F.

Place the purple yam in a baking pan with the cut side up.

Drizzle with 2/3 cup extra virgin olive oil, maple syrup , Italian seasoning and salt. Bake for 10 hours.

Drizzle with the remaining olive oil when you serve.

Cook's Note:

Do this overnight.

Roasted Carrots Parsnips and Turnips

Ingredients

3 medium carrots, sliced diagonally into chunks

3 medium parsnips, sliced diagonally into chunks

3 medium turnips, sliced diagonally into chunks

¾ cup sesame oil

3 tbsp. sesame seeds 2 tbsp. Sea Salt

2 tbsp. raw honey

Preheat the oven to 170 degrees F.

Place the vegetables in a baking pan with the cut side up.

Drizzle with 2/3 cup extra virgin olive oil, raw honey, Italian seasoning and salt. Bake for 10 hours.

Drizzle with the remaining olive oil when you serve.

Cook's Note:

Do this overnight.

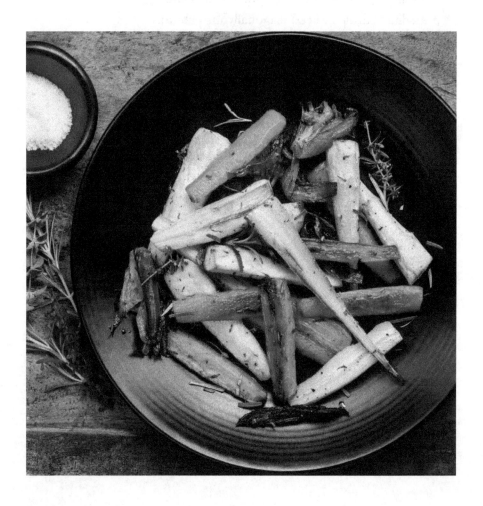

Bacon-wrapped Asparagus

Ingredients

1 ½ lbs. asparagus spears, trimmed 4 to 5 inches long tips Olive oil, for drizzling

A few pinches black pepper 4 slices bacon

Sea salt

Preheat the oven to 400 degrees F. Lightly coat the vegetables in olive oil. Season with salt and pepper, to taste.

Divide the vegetables and wrap with bacon/pancetta.

Do this for all of the vegetables and transfer to a greased cookie sheet.

Bake for 12 min

Crispy Fried Mahi Mahi fillet

Ingredients
2 pound Mahi-mahi fillets or strips 6 egg whites
2 1/2 cups almond flour Kosher salt

Add the egg whites to the almond flour and mix until smooth.
Dip the seafood into the batter and arrange them on a cookie sheet
Freeze them overnight.
Heat the deep fryer to 375 degrees F. Fry the seafood until pale gold in
color. Season with salt.

Fried Mackerel Fillet

Ingredients
2 pound Mackerel fillets or strips 6 egg whites
2 1/2 cups almond flour Kosher salt

Add the egg whites to the almond flour and mix until smooth.
Dip the seafood into the batter and arrange them on a cookie sheet
Freeze them overnight.
Heat the deep fryer to 375 degrees F. Fry the seafood until pale gold in color. Season with salt.

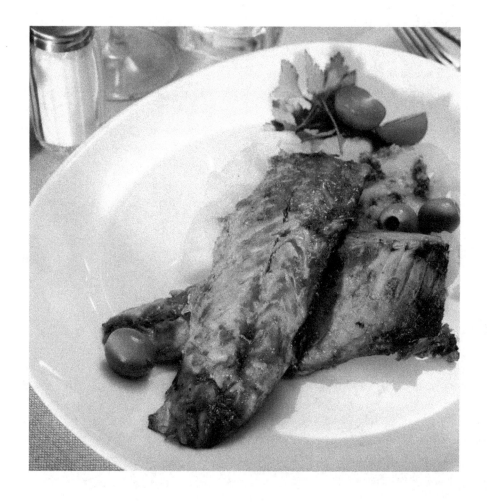

Striped Bass and Lime Ceviche

Ingredients

2 pound Striped bass fillets or strips 3 fresh kaffir lime leaves
Chopped fresh cilantro to taste 1 shallot, finely minced
Juice of 1 lime Juice of 1/2 lemon

Combine all of the ingredients and chill for one hour.

Scallops and Green Bell Pepper Ceviche

Ingredients

2 pounds scallops, shells removed 4 tomatoes, diced

5 green onions, minced 4 stalks celery, sliced

1 green bell pepper, minced 1 cup chopped fresh parsley freshly ground black pepper

4 tablespoons extra virgin olive oil

Combine all of the ingredients and chill for one hour.

Perfectly Fried Eggs

Ingredients

1 really fresh large egg

2 tablespoons organic butter Pinch of sea salt

2-3 drops balsamic vinegar (optional) 1 tbsp. Water

Preheat the oven to 475 degrees Fahrenheit.

Break the egg carefully and separate the white from the yolk. Make sure that yours does not break.

Add the butter and the water to the frying pan and heat until foaming.

Add salt to the pan so that the egg whites get seasoned

As the butter starts to foam, slide in the egg white.

Take it out of the heat and put it in the oven for 1 ½ minutes. Season with salt and add the raw yolk and bake for 2 more minutes. Add some drops of

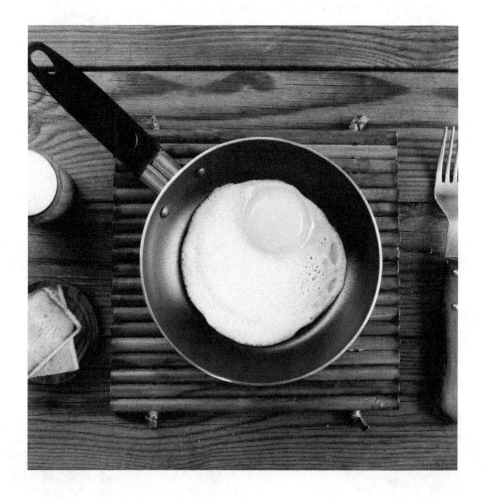

Perfectly Poached Eggs

Ingredients
1 fresh large eggs Few drops of vinegar Pinch of sea salt Water to boil

Crack the eggs and add a few drops of white wine vinegar. Boil the water in a pan and stir it in a circular motion.
Add the eggs to the water as it's swirling and turn off the heat. Leave it there for 4 to 5 minutes and lift it out with a slotted spoon.

Shrimp and Bell Pepper Stuffed Avocado

Ingredients

½ medium avocado 3 large eggs

Pinch of kosher salt

1 tbsp. Sliced jalapenos 4 tbsp. Nutritional Yeast 3 tsp. Tajin seasoning

1 tbsp. Extra virgin olive oil Spice Ingredients

1 tsp. chili powder 1 tsp. Onion powder

½ tsp. garlic powder

¼ cup cashew cheese Filling Ingredients

3 ounces shrimp, peeled and deveined 3 ounces carrots, diced

5 ounces eggplant diced

1/2 medium green bell pepper diced

Preheat the oven to 400 degrees F.

Spread all of the filling ingredients and drizzle with olive oil.

Add all of the seasoning ingredients except the cashew cheese and toss to coat. Layer evenly.

Bake for 10 to 15 min. until browned.

Take the vegetables out and top with the cashew cheese. Sliced the avocado in half and take out the seed.

Place the vegetables inside the pit of the avocado.

Add the vegetable mixture and crack the eggs on top of the mixture.

Bake for 10 min.

Top with jalapenos, cashew cheese and tajin.

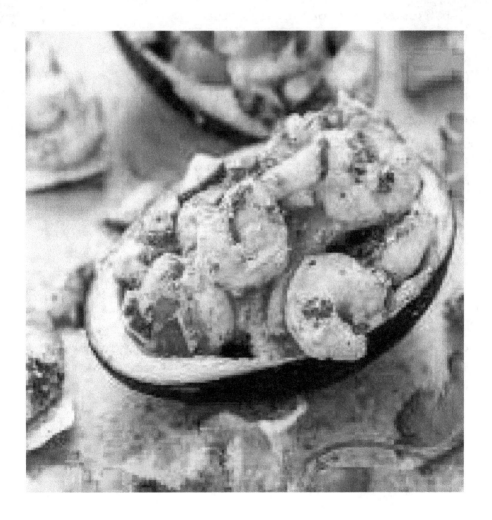

Sole Fish Fillet and Eggplant Stuffed Avocado

Ingredients

½ medium avocado 3 large eggs

Pinch of sea salt

1 tbsp. Sliced jalapenos 4 tbsp. Nutritional Yeast 3 tsp. Tajin seasoning

1 tbsp. Extra virgin olive oil Spice Ingredients

1 tsp. Greek seasoning 1 tsp. Onion powder

½ tsp. garlic powder

¼ cup cashew cheese Filling Ingredients

3 ounces sole fish fillet, sliced into small chunks 3 ounces carrots, diced

5 ounces eggplant diced

1/2 medium green bell pepper diced

Preheat the oven to 400 degrees F.

Spread all of the filling ingredients and drizzle with olive oil.

Add all of the seasoning ingredients except the cashew cheese and toss
to coat. Layer evenly.

Bake for 10 to 15 min. until browned.

Take the vegetables out and top with the cashew cheese. Sliced the
avocado in half and take out the seed.

Place the vegetables inside the pit of the avocado.

Add the vegetable mixture and crack the eggs on top of the mixture.

Bake for 10 min.

Top with jalapenos, cashew cheese and tajin.

Paleo Frittata

Ingredients
Olive oil
1 green bell pepper
8 slices of smoking bacon
3 spring onions sliced diagonally Handful basil
⅔ lbs. Frozen peas
4 ½ ounces of cashew cheese 8 eggs beaten
¼ cup grated nutritional yeast Black pepper
Pinch of sea salt

Preheat oven to 350 degrees Heat the olive oil in a frying pan
Add the bacon and fry for 2 ½ minutes
Add the bell pepper and cook until bacon turns golden brown. Add the spring onions and cook for 4 to 5 minutes until it's tender Add the peas.
Sprinkle some basil.
Top with 2 ½ ounces of chunks of cashew cheese. Heat your broiler to the highest setting.
Combine the beaten eggs nutritional yeast, sea salt and black pepper in a bowl. Pour this mixture over the cooked vegetables and bacon.
Shake the pan over medium heat until the omelet sets at the bottom.
Crumble the remaining cottage cheese.
Place the pain under the broiler for 4 ½ minutes. Slide frittata out of the pan and cut into wedges.

Pan-fried Chicken Breast with Caramelized Onion

Ingredients

1 tbsp. Extra virgin olive oil
4 pcs. Of 4-ounce ½-inch thick boneless chicken breast 1 onion cut into strips
1 cup water

Seasoning mixture
½ tsp. Sea salt
½ tsp. Italian Seasoning
½ tsp. Garlic powder
¼ tsp. Onion powder

Combine all of the ingredients for the seasoning mixture. Rub it all over the meat.

Heat a skillet in medium high heat. Brown the meat while flipping it often. Add the onions and water to the pan.

Reduce the heat and simmer for 20 min.

Turn the meat and cook until water evaporates and onions turn light to medium brown. Remove the meat and top with the onions.

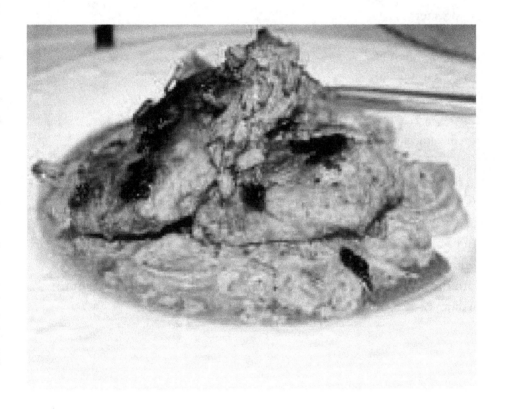

Pan-fried Garlic Duck Breast

Ingredients
1 tbsp. Extra virgin olive oil
4 pcs. Of 4-ounce ½-inch thick boneless duck breast 1 onion cut into strips
1 cup water

Seasoning mixture
½ tsp. Kosher salt
½ tsp. Greek Seasoning
½ tsp. Garlic powder
¼ tsp. Onion powder

Combine all of the ingredients for the seasoning mixture. Rub it all over the meat.
Heat a skillet in medium high heat. Brown the meat while flipping it often. Add the onions and water to the pan.
Reduce the heat and simmer for 20 min.
Turn the meat and cook until water evaporates and onions turn light to medium brown. Remove the meat and top with the onions.

Spicy Roasted Sirloin

Ingredients
4 slices 1-inch thick Sirloin
¼ cup extra virgin olive oil 2 tsp. Salt
Spice Ingredients
1 tsp. Garlic powder 1 tsp. Onion powder
1 tsp. Cayenne Pepper

Preheat the oven to 400 degrees F
Grease the baking sheet and rub each meat with oil.
Combine the spice ingredients and season all sides of the meat with this mixture.
Place the meat in the baking sheet and bake for 18 min. or until it reaches an internal temperature of 145 degrees F.
Notes: Make sure to take them out at 145 degrees F so you don't lose too much moisture.

Smoky Roasted Tenderloin

Ingredients

4 slices 1-inch thick tenderloin roast

¼ cup extra virgin olive oil 2 tsp. Salt

Spice Ingredients 1 tsp. Cumin

1 tsp. Onion powder

1 tsp. Smoked paprika

Preheat the oven to 400 degrees F

Grease the baking sheet and rub each meat with oil.

Combine the spice ingredients and season all sides of the meat with this mixture.

Place the meat in the baking sheet and bake for 18 min. or until it reaches an internal temperature of 145 degrees F.

Notes: Make sure to take them out at 145 degrees F so you don't lose too much moisture.

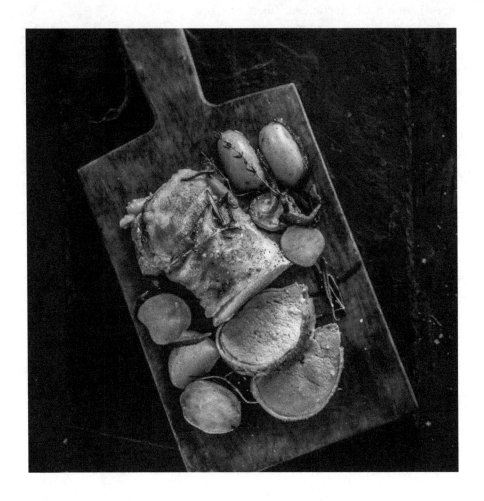

Roasted Arctic Char Fillet with Rainbow Peppercorns

Ingredients

4 slices 1-inch thick Arctic char fillets or strips

¼ cup extra virgin olive oil 2 tsp. Salt

Spice Ingredients

1 tsp. Garlic powder 1 tsp. Onion powder

1 tsp. Rainbow Peppercorns

Preheat the oven to 400 degrees F

Grease the baking sheet and rub each fish with oil.

Combine the spice ingredients and season all sides of the fish with this mixture.

Place the fish in the baking sheet and bake for 18 min. or until it reaches an internal temperature of 145 degrees F.

Notes: Make sure to take them out at 145 degrees F so you don't lose too much moisture.

Italian-Style Roasted Flounder Fillet

Ingredients

4 slices 1-inch thick Flounder fillets or strips

¼ cup extra virgin olive oil 2 tsp. Salt

Spice Ingredients

1 tsp. Garlic powder 1 tsp. Onion powder

1 tsp. Italian Seasoning

Preheat the oven to 400 degrees F

Grease the baking sheet and rub each fish with oil.

Combine the spice ingredients and season all sides of the fish with this mixture.

Place the fish in the baking sheet and bake for 18 min. or until it reaches an internal temperature of 145 degrees F.

Notes: Make sure to take them out at 145 degrees F so you don't lose too much moisture.

Beef Strip loin Stuffed Eggplants

Ingredients
2 large eggplants 4 tbsp. olive oil
3 ounces nutritional yeast, shredded 1 cup cauliflower florets
6 ounces beef strip loin, sliced thinly
2 tbsp. Sour cream/ dairy free sour cream 1 stalk green onion
Sea salt, to taste

Preheat the oven to 400 degrees F
Cut the zucchini/eggplant lengthwise and use a melon baller to scoop out the middle.
Pour 1 tbsp. oil into each zucchini/eggplant and season with salt and pepper and bake for 20 min. Stir fry the meat on medium high heat. Stir often until browned.
Cut the florets into small pieces.
Blanch the florets by dipping them into boiling water for 2 min.
Combine the florets and meat with the sour cream.
As the zucchini/eggplant finishes baking, add the meat and vegetable filling.
Sprinkle the nutritional yeast and bake for 10 to 15 min. or until the nutritional yeast browns. Garnish with the finely chopped green onion.

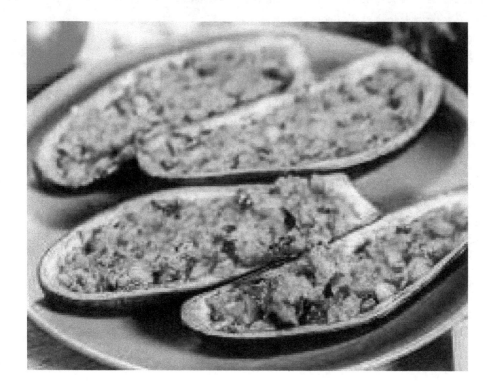

Chicken Breast and Cauliflower Stuffed Eggplants

Ingredients
2 large eggplants 4 tbsp. Sesame oil
3 ounces nutritional yeast, shredded 1 cup cauliflower florets
6 ounces chicken breast fillet, sliced thinly 2 tbsp. Sour cream/ dairy
free sour cream 1 stalk green onion
Sea salt, to taste

Preheat the oven to 400 degrees F
Cut the zucchini/eggplant lengthwise and use a melon baller to scoop out the middle.
Pour 1 tbsp. oil into each zucchini/eggplant and season with salt and pepper and bake for 20 min. Stir fry the meat on medium high heat. Stir often until browned.
Cut the florets into small pieces.
Blanch the florets by dipping them into boiling water for 2 min.
Combine the florets and meat with the sour cream.
As the zucchini/eggplant finishes baking, add the meat and vegetable filling.
Sprinkle the nutritional yeast and bake for 10 to 15 min. or until the nutritional yeast browns. Garnish with the finely chopped green onion.

Chicken Breast Fillet and Cauliflower Stuffed Zucchini with Sour Cream

Ingredients

2 large zucchini 4 tbsp. olive oil
3 ounces nutritional yeast, shredded 1 cup cauliflower florets
6 ounces chicken breast fillet, sliced thinly 2 tbsp. Sour cream/ dairy free sour cream 1 stalk green onion
Sea salt, to taste

Preheat the oven to 400 degrees F
Cut the zucchini/eggplant lengthwise and use a melon baller to scoop out the middle.
Pour 1 tbsp. oil into each zucchini/eggplant and season with salt and pepper and bake for 20 min. Stir fry the meat on medium high heat. Stir often until browned.
Cut the florets into small pieces.
Blanch the florets by dipping them into boiling water for 2 min.
Combine the florets and meat with the sour cream.
As the zucchini/eggplant finishes baking, add the meat and vegetable filling.
Sprinkle the nutritional yeast and bake for 10 to 15 min. or until the nutritional yeast browns. Garnish with the finely chopped green onion.

Pork Loin and Broccoli Stuffed Eggplants

Ingredients

2 large eggplants 4 tbsp. Sesame oil

3 ounces nutritional yeast, shredded 1 cup broccoli florets

6 ounces pork loin, sliced thinly

2 tbsp. Sour cream/ dairy free sour cream 1 stalk green onion

Sea salt, to taste

Preheat the oven to 400 degrees F

Cut the zucchini/eggplant lengthwise and use a melon baller to scoop out the middle.

Pour 1 tbsp. oil into each zucchini/eggplant and season with salt and pepper and bake for 20 min. Stir fry the meat on medium high heat. Stir often until browned.

Cut the florets into small pieces.

Blanch the florets by dipping them into boiling water for 2 min.

Combine the florets and meat with the sour cream.

As the zucchini/eggplant finishes baking, add the meat and vegetable filling.

Sprinkle the nutritional yeast and bake for 10 to 15 min. or until the nutritional yeast browns. Garnish with the finely chopped green onion.

Mixed Greens and Bacon with Balsamic Mayonnaise

Base Salad Ingredients 2 ¼ oz mixed greens 1/4 cup pine nuts
2 slices of bacon
2 tbsp. Nutritional Yeast
Dressing Ingredients
1 tbsp. Mayonnaise (no soybean oil) 1 tbsp. Balsamic Vinegar
1 tsp. Sour cream
2 tbsp. Extra virgin olive oil 1/2 tsp. sesame seeds
Sea salt

Combine all of the dressing ingredients Combine all of the base salad ingredients Cut the bacon into squares.
Cook the bacon until brown and crisp over medium high heat.
Crumble them on top of the salad ingredients
Drizzle with vinaigrette

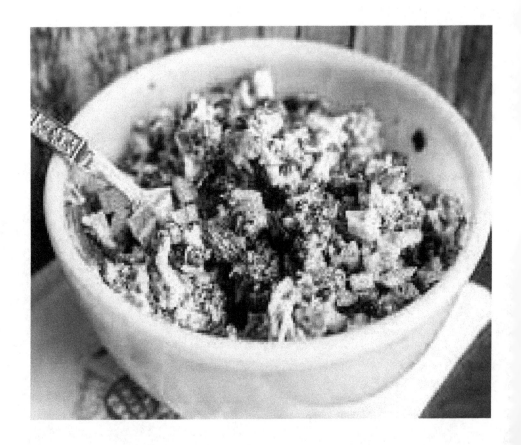

Romaine Lettuce with Pine Nuts and Sour Cream Dressing

Base Salad Ingredients 2 ¼ oz Romaine Lettuce 1/4 cup pine nuts
2 slices of bacon
2 tbsp. Nutritional Yeast
Dressing Ingredients
1 tbsp. Mayonnaise (no soybean oil) 1 tbsp. White Wine Vinegar
1 tsp. Sour cream 2 tbsp. olive oil
1/2 tsp. Greek seasoning Sea salt

Combine all of the dressing ingredients Combine all of the base salad ingredients Cut the bacon into squares.
Cook the bacon until brown and crisp over medium high heat.
Crumble them on top of the salad ingredients
Drizzle with vinaigrette

Romaine Lettuce with Pine Nuts and Bacon Salad

Base Salad Ingredients 2 ¼ oz Romaine Lettuce 1/4 cup pine nuts
1 slices of bacon
2 tbsp. Nutritional Yeast
Dressing Ingredients
1 tbsp. Mayonnaise (no soybean oil) 1 tbsp. Red Wine Vinegar
1 tsp. Sour cream
2 tbsp. Extra virgin olive oil 1/2 tsp. Greek seasoning Sea salt
Combine all of the dressing ingredients Combine all of the base salad
ingredients Cut the bacon into squares.
Cook the bacon until brown and crisp over medium high heat.
Crumble them on top of the salad ingredients
Drizzle with vinaigrette

Ice Berg Lettuce with Bacon and Walnuts

Base Salad Ingredients 2 ¼ oz Iceberg Lettuce 1/4 cup walnuts
2 slices of bacon
2 tbsp. Nutritional Yeast
Dressing Ingredients
1 tbsp. Mayonnaise (no soybean oil) 1 tbsp. Balsamic Vinegar
1 tsp. Dijon Mustard
2 tbsp. Extra virgin olive oil 1/2 tsp. sesame seeds
Sea salt

Combine all of the dressing ingredients Combine all of the base salad
ingredients Cut the bacon into squares.
Cook the bacon until brown and crisp over medium high heat.
Crumble them on top of the salad ingredients
Drizzle with vinaigrette

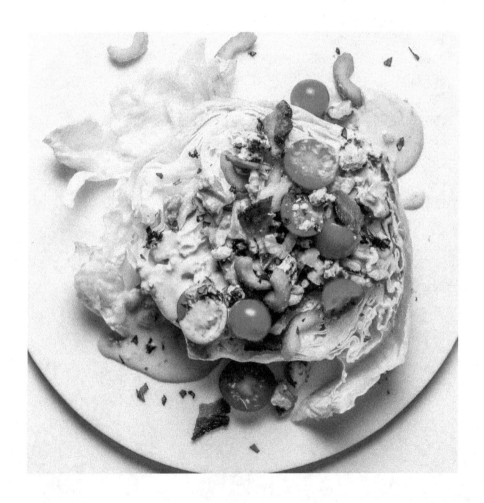

Spicy Sirloin and Chuck Meatballs

Main Ingredients
½ pound ground sirloin
½ pound ground chuck
1 medium red onions, chopped
½ medium yellow bell pepper 2 tbsp. Cilantro, finely chopped
½ tsp. Onion powder
½ tsp. Chili Powder
½ tsp. Sea Salt
½ tsp. Red pepper flakes
Juice and zest of ¼ medium lemon 2 ounces cashew cheese
2 tbsp. Flaxseed meal 2 tbsp. Almond flour

Guacamole
1 medium avocado
Juice of ⅓ of medium lime 1 tbsp. finely minced garlic Sea Salt
Extra virgin olive oil

Preheat the oven to 350 degrees F.
Combine all of the main ingredients together. Roll them into meatballs
and bake for 18 min. Combine all of the guacamole ingredients.
Serve the meatballs with guacamole.

Smoky Beef and Lamb Meatballs

Main Ingredients
½ pound ground beef
½ pound ground lamb
2 medium red onions, chopped
½ medium green bell pepper
2 tbsp. Cilantro, finely chopped
½ tsp. cumin
½ tsp. Garlic powder
½ tsp. Sea Salt
½ tsp. Red pepper flakes
Juice and zest of ¼ medium lime 2 ounces cashew cheese
2 tbsp. Flaxseed meal 2 tbsp. Almond flour

Guacamole
1 medium avocado
Juice of ⅓ of medium lime 1 tbsp. finely minced garlic Sea Salt
Extra virgin olive oil

Preheat the oven to 350 degrees F.
Combine all of the main ingredients together. Roll them into meatballs and bake for 18 min. Combine all of the guacamole ingredients.
Serve the meatballs with guacamole.

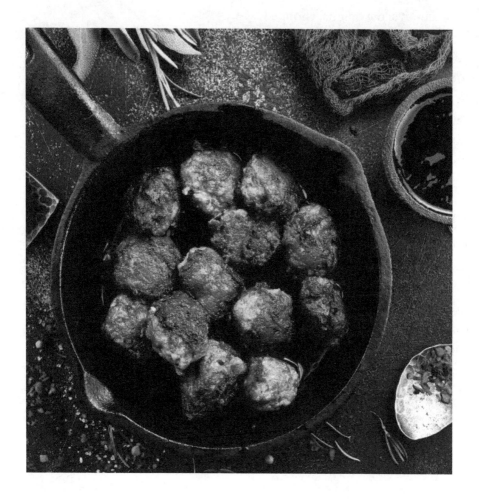

Smoky Lamb Bell Pepper and Beef Meatballs

Main Ingredients
½ pound ground beef
½ pound ground lamb
2 medium yellow onions, chopped
½ medium yellow bell pepper 2 tbsp. Cilantro, finely chopped
½ tsp. cumin
½ tsp. chili powder
½ tsp. Sea Salt
½ tsp. Red pepper flakes
Juice and zest of ¼ medium lemon 2 ounces cashew cheese
2 tbsp. Flaxseed meal 2 tbsp. Almond flour

Guacamole
1 medium avocado
Juice of ⅓ of medium lime 1 tbsp. finely minced garlic Sea Salt
Extra virgin olive oil

Preheat the oven to 350 degrees F.
Combine all of the main ingredients together. Roll them into meatballs
and bake for 18 min. Combine all of the guacamole ingredients.
Serve the meatballs with guacamole.

Bib Lettuce with Tomato and Sesame Dressing

Salad Ingredients

4 Slices of bacon, cut into squares 2 cups bib lettuce

¼ cup cilantro, chopped finely

¼ medium green bell pepper, chopped

Sauce Ingredients 2 tbsp. Tomato paste 3 tbsp. sea salt

1 tbsp. Sesame oil

1 tbsp. chili garlic paste 2 tbsp. Chopped cilantro

½ tsp. sesame seeds Juice & zest of ½ lime

¼ tsp. Sichuan peppercorns 4 tsp. apple cider vinegar

½ tsp. Red pepper flakes 1 tsp. Fish sauce

2 tbsp. raw honey

Over medium heat, fry the bacon until brown and crisp over medium heat. Combine the salad ingredients.

Combine all of the sauce ingredients.

Toss the salad with the sauce ingredients and top with the bacon

Lettuce and Bacon with Pesto and Tomato Dressing

Salad Ingredients
4 Slices of bacon, cut into squares 2 cups iceberg lettuce
¼ cup cilantro, chopped finely
¼ medium yellow bell pepper, chopped
Sauce Ingredients 2 tbsp. Tomato paste 3 tbsp. sea salt
2 tbsp. olive oil 1 tbsp. Pesto
2 tbsp. Chopped parsley 1 tsp. mustard
Juice & zest of ½ lemon 4 tsp. apple cider vinegar
½ tsp. Red pepper flakes

Over medium heat, fry the bacon until brown and crisp over medium heat. Combine the salad ingredients.
Combine all of the sauce ingredients.
Toss the salad with the sauce ingredients and top with the bacon

Mustard Greens and Turnip Greens Curry

Ingredients
Vegetable Ingredients
½ cup broccoli florets
½ cup mustard greens
1 large handful of turnip greens 4 tbsp. Extra virgin coconut oil
¼ medium onion
Aromatic Ingredients
1 tsp. Thai bird chilies, minced 1 tsp. Minced garlic
1 tsp. Minced ginger 3 tsp. Fish sauce
1 tsp. Soy sauce
½ tsp. Sea salt
1 tbsp. Green curry paste 1 tbsp. Sriracha
½ cup coconut milk

Chopped onions and minced garlic
Add 2 tbsp. Coconut oil and cook over medium heat. Add onions and cook until translucent
Add the garlic and cook until golden brown. Turn the heat to medium-low and add the florets.
Keep stirring until the florets are partially cooked. Add the rest of the aromatic ingredients.
Cook for 1 more minute.
Add the remaining vegetable ingredients, coconut cream and coconut oil. Stir together and simmer for 5 to 10 min.

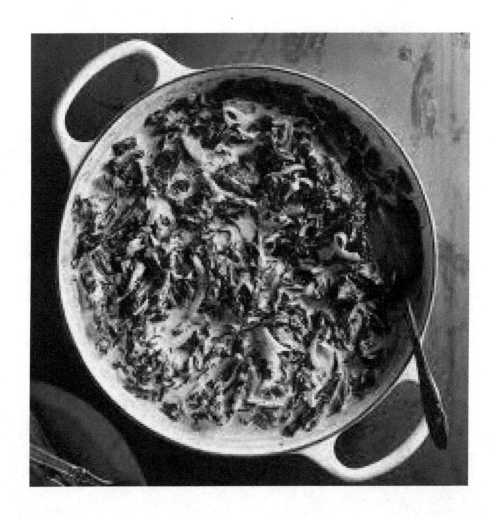

Beet Greens and Kale Curry

Ingredients

Vegetable Ingredients 3/4 cup broccoli florets 1/4 cup kale
1 large handful of beet greens 4 tbsp. Extra virgin coconut oil
¼ medium red onion
Aromatic Ingredients 1/2 tsp. cumin
1 tsp. Minced garlic 1 tsp. Minced ginger 3 tsp. Fish sauce
1 tsp. Soy sauce
½ tsp. Sea salt
1 tbsp. red curry paste 1 tbsp. Sriracha
½ cup coconut milk

Chopped onions and minced garlic
Add 2 tbsp. Coconut oil and cook over medium heat. Add onions and cook until translucent
Add the garlic and cook until golden brown. Turn the heat to medium-low and add the florets.
Keep stirring until the florets are partially cooked. Add the rest of the aromatic ingredients.
Cook for 1 more minute.
Add the remaining vegetable ingredients, coconut cream and coconut oil. Stir together and simmer for 5 to 10 min.

Sirloin and Sun-dried Tomato Patty

Ingredients

12 ounces ground sirloin 4 slices bacon

2 medium Sweet Italian peppers

¼ cup sun-dried tomato pesto

¼ cup nutritional yeast 1 large egg

3 tbsp. sesame seeds Pinch of sea salt

Fry the bacon until brown and crisp on medium-high heat.

In a food processor, chop the bell peppers and take out the moisture with the paper towel. Put the meat and bacon in the food processor and blend until smooth.

Add and combine this with the rest of the ingredients thoroughly.

Form into patties and fry in medium heat until golden brown.

Duck and Sun-dried Tomato Pesto Patty

Ingredients

12 ounces duck breast, deboned and chopped 4 slices bacon

2 medium Sweet Italian peppers

¼ cup sun-dried tomato pesto

¼ cup cashew cheese 1 large egg

3 tbsp. Almond flour Pinch of sea salt

Fry the bacon until brown and crisp on medium-high heat.

In a food processor, chop the bell peppers and take out the moisture with the paper towel. Put the meat and bacon in the food processor and blend until smooth.

Add and combine this with the rest of the ingredients thoroughly.

Form into patties and fry in medium heat until golden brown.

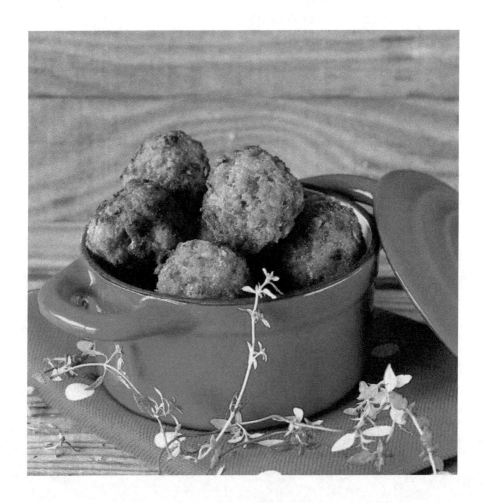

Asian Roast Chicken Red Onion Lettuce Wraps

Ingredients

half a pound leftover roast chicken

½ tsp. sesame seeds 6 pcs. Butter lettuce

⅓ Green Bell Pepper, sliced into thin strips

¼ Medium Red Onion, sliced into thin strips 2 tsp. Garlic Chili Paste

1 tsp. Sesame oil

½ tsp. sesame seeds

½ tsp. Red Pepper Flakes Sea Salt and pepper to taste

Debone the meat.

Shred the meat into small pieces.

Combine the meat with the rest of the ingredients and place them on a piece of butter lettuce. Add some salt and pepper.

Drizzle with sesame seeds Roll the lettuce up.

Chili Garlic Roast Chicken in Lettuce Wraps

Ingredients
half a pound leftover roast turkey
½ tsp. sesame seeds 6 pcs. Butter lettuce
2 Sweet Italian Peppers, sliced into thin strips
¼ Medium Red Onion, sliced into thin strips 2 tsp. Garlic Chili Paste
1 tbsp. almond butter 1 tsp. Peanut oil
½ tsp. sesame seeds
½ tsp. Cayenne Pepper
Sea Salt and pepper to taste

Debone the meat.
Shred the meat into small pieces.
Combine the meat with the rest of the ingredients and place them on a piece of butter lettuce. Add some salt and pepper.
Drizzle with sesame seeds Roll the lettuce up.

Sirloin and Pork Burger in Portobello Bread

Ingredients
1 tbsp. olive oil
1 clove garlic, minced 1 tsp. Italian seasoning
¼ tsp. Sea salt
¼ tsp. Rainbow Peppercorns
2 caps Portobello mushroom caps
Burger Patty
3 ounces ground beef sirloin 3 ounces ground pork
1 tbsp. Dijon mustard 1 tsp. Sea salt.
¼ cup cashew cheese

Combine oil, salt and spices
Clean the mushrooms by taking out the gills. Marinate them with the oil and the spices
To make the patty, combine all of the burger patty ingredients. Form them into a round patty.
Place the Portobello mushrooms on the grill and cook for 8 min. Add the burger to the grill and cook for 5 min. on each side.
Top with cashew cheese.
Assemble the burger by placing it in between the Portobello mushrooms.

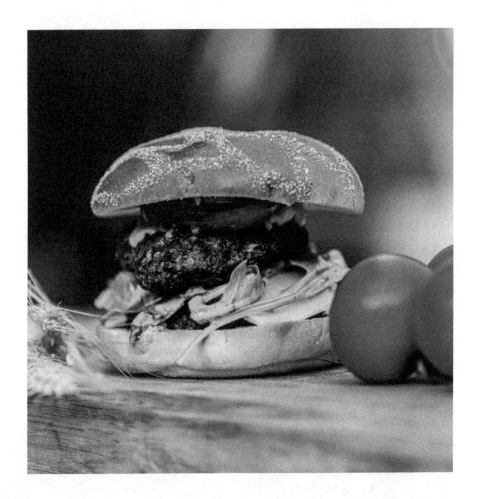

Chicken Burger in Portobello Bread with Cashew Cheese

Ingredients
1 tbsp. olive oil

1 clove garlic, minced 1 tsp. Greek seasoning

¼ tsp. Sea salt

¼ tsp. Rainbow Peppercorns

2 caps Portobello mushroom caps

Burger Patty

6 ounces ground chicken thighs 1 egg

1 tsp. Sea salt.

¼ cup cashew cheese

Combine oil, salt and spices

Clean the mushrooms by taking out the gills. Marinate them with the oil and the spices

To make the patty, combine all of the burger patty ingredients. Form them into a round patty.

Place the Portobello mushrooms on the grill and cook for 8 min. Add the burger to the grill and cook for 5 min. on each side.

Top with cashew cheese.

Assemble the burger by placing it in between the Portobello mushrooms.

Pan-fried Pollock Fillet

Ingredients Dredging Ingredients Sea salt, to taste
Coconut Flour for dredging Main Ingredients
1 large Pollock fillet 2 tbsp. Olive oil
3 tbsp. Butter Garnishing Ingredients 1 tbsp. Capers, drained Juice of 1
lemon

Season the fish with salt
Coat the fish with the remaining dredging ingredients. Heat the butter
with the olive oil.
As soon as it starts to foam, place fish skin-side down. Jiggle the pan to
keep the skin from sticking. Cook until a crust forms. Flip the fish and
jiggle for a few seconds once more to keep it from sticking.
Cook until golden brown.
Fry the garnishing ingredients except the juice with the remaining fat
Sprinkle with juice once it's finished.
Pour the sauce over the fish.

Pan-fried Arctic Char Fillet

Ingredients Dredging Ingredients Sea salt, to taste
1 cup Almond flour for dredging 1/2 tsp. Cayenne Pepper
Main Ingredients
1 large Arctic char fillet 2 tbsp. Olive oil
3 tbsp. Butter Garnishing Ingredients 1 tbsp. Capers, drained Juice of 1
lemon

Season the fish with salt
Coat the fish with the remaining dredging ingredients. Heat the butter
with the olive oil.
As soon as it starts to foam, place fish skin-side down. Jiggle the pan to
keep the skin from sticking. Cook until a crust forms. Flip the fish and
jiggle for a few seconds once more to keep it from sticking.
Cook until golden brown.
Fry the garnishing ingredients except the juice with the remaining fat
Sprinkle with juice once it's finished.
Pour the sauce over the fish.

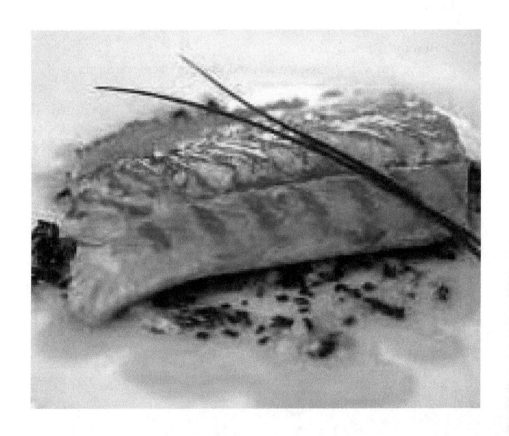

Roasted Italian Garlic Chicken

Ingredients

8 turkey breast Seasoning Ingredients
¾ cup extra virgin olive oil 2 tsp. Italian Seasoning
40 peeled cloves of garlic Sea Salt

Preheat the oven 350 degrees F. Generously season the meat with salt.
In a skillet, pan fry meat with olive oil on medium high heat. Take it
out of the heat and add seasoning ingredients.
Place them in a baking pan and cover. Bake for 1 ½ hours.
Let them rest for 5 to 10 min. Carve and serve.

Asian Roasted Chili Garlic Pheasant

Ingredients

1 Whole Pheasant Quartered Seasoning Ingredients

¾ cup extra virgin olive oil 2 tbsp. chili powder

40 peeled cloves of garlic Sea Salt

Preheat the oven 350 degrees F. Generously season the meat with salt. In a skillet, pan fry meat with olive oil on medium high heat. Take it out of the heat and add seasoning ingredients.

Place them in a baking pan and cover. Bake for 1 ½ hours.

Let them rest for 5 to 10 min. Carve and serve.

Haddock Fillet Cakes and Capers

Ingredients
1/2 pound Haddock fillets
¾ cup Olive oil
Sea salt and pepper, to taste Aromatic Ingredients
¾ cup diced red onion 1 cup diced celery
1 cup green bell pepper
½ cup yellow bell pepper
¼ cup flat-leaf parsley, minced 2 tsp. Capers
¼ tsp. Tabasco
½ tsp. Worcestershire sauce 1 ½ tsp. Old bay seasoning Binding
Ingredients
1 cup almond flour
½ cup mayonnaise
2 tsp. English mustard
2 large eggs, lightly beaten

Preheat the oven to 350 degrees F
Place the fish skin-side down on a sheet pan and brush with olive oil.
Sprinkle some salt and pepper and roast for 15 to 20 minutes.
Take it out of the oven and rest for 10 min.
Over medium low-heat, add the aromatic ingredients Cook until
vegetables are tender.
Toast the almond flour by spreading it evenly on a baking sheet and
roasting it in the oven for 5 min.
Flake the fish in a large bowl and combine with all of the seasoning and
binding ingredients. Chill in the refrigerator for 30 minutes.
Shape them into 10 pcs. of 3-ounce cakes.
Heat the remaining butter and olive oil over medium heat.
Fry the fish cakes for 3 to 4 minutes on each side until browned. Drain
and bake in the oven at 250 degrees F.
Rest for 2 min. and serve.

Snapper Fillet and Green Olive Fish Cakes

Ingredients
1/2 pound Snapper fillets
¾ cup Olive oil
Sea salt and pepper, to taste Aromatic Ingredients
¾ cup diced white onion
1 ½ cups yellow bell pepper
¼ cup flat-leaf parsley, minced 2 tsp. Green Olives
¼ tsp. Tabasco
½ tsp. Worcestershire sauce 1 ½ tsp. Old bay seasoning Binding
Ingredients
1 cup almond flour
½ cup mayonnaise
2 tsp. English mustard
2 large eggs, lightly beaten

Preheat the oven to 350 degrees F
Place the fish skin-side down on a sheet pan and brush with olive oil.
Sprinkle some salt and pepper and roast for 15 to 20 minutes.
Take it out of the oven and rest for 10 min.
Over medium low-heat, add the aromatic ingredients Cook until
vegetables are tender.
Toast the almond flour by spreading it evenly on a baking sheet and
roasting it in the oven for 5 min.
Flake the fish in a large bowl and combine with all of the seasoning and
binding ingredients. Chill in the refrigerator for 30 minutes.
Shape them into 10 pcs. of 3-ounce cakes.
Heat the remaining butter and olive oil over medium heat.
Fry the fish cakes for 3 to 4 minutes on each side until browned. Drain
and bake in the oven at 250 degrees F.
Rest for 2 min. and serve.

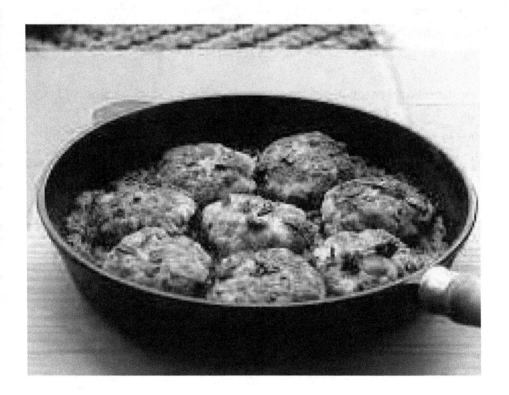

Beef Spinach and Red Onion Chili

Ingredients

4 tbsp. extra virgin olive oil 1 medium red onion, diced 2 lbs. ground chuck

3 ¾ cups chicken broth 3 cups coconut cream 3 tbsp. lemon juice
Aromatic Ingredients

11 ounces diced Sweet Italian Peppers 2 tsp. Sea salt

1 tsp. Cumin

½ tsp oregano

1 tsp. Black pepper 1/4 lb. frozen spinach

Heat the oil over medium heat in a pressure cooker. Add the onion and meat.

Cook until the onion becomes tender.

Add the aromatic ingredients to the mixture Stir and add 4 cups of broth.

Cover and cook for 30 minutes at high pressure. Let it sit for 10 min. before releasing the steam.

Pork & Broccoli Chili

Ingredients

4 tbsp. extra virgin olive oil 1 medium red onion, diced 2 lbs. ground pork

3 ¾ cups chicken broth 3 cups coconut cream 3 tbsp. lemon juice

Aromatic Ingredients

10 ounces diced New Mexico Chilies 2 tsp. Sea salt

1 tsp. paprika

½ tsp oregano

1 tsp. Black pepper 1 lb. frozen broccoli

Heat the oil over medium heat in a pressure cooker. Add the onion and meat.

Cook until the onion becomes tender.

Add the aromatic ingredients to the mixture Stir and add 4 cups of broth.

Cover and cook for 30 minutes at high pressure. Let it sit for 10 min. before releasing the steam.

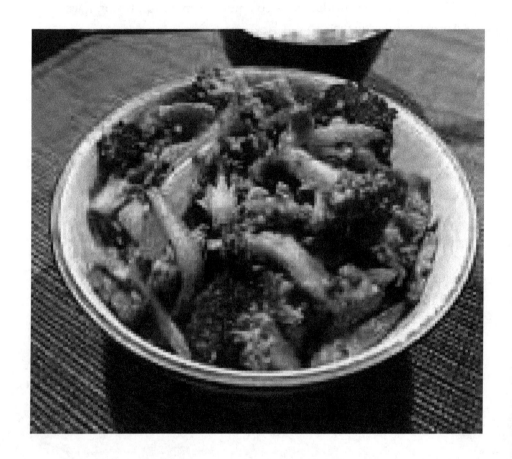

Fried Perch Fillets

Ingredients

7 ounces Perch fillets or strips 4 tbsp. extra virgin olive oil

2 tbsp. Lemon juice

Dredging Ingredients

2 tbsp. coarsely ground almonds 1/4 cup almond flour

1 tsp. Cayenne Pepper 1 tsp. Smoked Paprika 1 tsp. Garlic powder

½ tsp. Onion powder Sea Salt to taste

Combine the dredging ingredients thoroughly. Take the fillets and coat them with this mixture.

Heat the oil and add the lemon juice over medium-high heat. Sear the fish for 3 minutes on each side.

Make sure to swirl the pan to keep the fish from sticking. Do not overcook the fish.

Fried Rainbow Trout Fillets

Ingredients

7 ounces Rainbow trout fillets or strips 4 tbsp. extra virgin olive oil

2 tbsp. Lemon juice

Dredging Ingredients

¼ cup almond flour 2 tbsp. flax meal

1 tsp. marjoram

1 tsp. chili powder 1 tsp. Garlic powder

½ tsp. Onion powder Sea Salt to taste

Combine the dredging ingredients thoroughly. Take the fillets and coat them with this mixture.

Heat the oil and add the lemon juice over medium-high heat. Sear the fish for 3 minutes on each side.

Make sure to swirl the pan to keep the fish from sticking. Do not overcook the fish.

Barbecued Baby Back Ribs

Ingredients

3 lb. baby back ribs 1 cup pork broth

¼ cup apple cider vinegar 2 tsp. Liquid smoke

Rub Ingredients

1 tbsp. Paprika

1 ½ tsp. Garlic powder 1 ½ tsp. Onion powder 1 ½ tsp. Black pepper

½ tsp. Chili powder 1 ½ tsp. Cumin

¼ tsp. Cayenne pepper 1 tsp. Sea salt

½ tsp. Dry mustard

Barbecue Sauce

1 ½ cup mayonnaise

¼ cup apple cider vinegar 1 tbsp. English mustard

1 tsp. Black pepper 1 tsp. Salt

3 tsp. garlic , minced 2 tbsp. raw honey

2   tsp. Prepared horseradish

Combine all of the rub ingredients thoroughly.

Wash and dry the meat and take out any silver skin using a sharp knife. Season the meat thoroughly with the rub mixture until the entire surface is coated.

Add the pork broth, apple cider vinegar and liquid smoke into the pressure cooker together with the meat and cook on high for 35 min. Release the steam.

Combine all the sauce ingredients in a bowl and let it rest in the refrigerator for 3 hours. Preheat the oven to 450 degrees F.

Roast the meat for 6 minutes on each side or until crisp.

Barbecued Beef Brisket

Ingredients

3 lbs. beef brisket 1 cup pork broth

¼ cup apple cider vinegar 2 tsp. Liquid smoke

Rub Ingredients

1 tbsp. Raw Honey

1 ½ tsp. Garlic powder 1 ½ tsp. Onion powder

1 ½ tsp. Finely Ground Coffee Beans

½ tsp. Smoked Paprika 1 ½ tsp. Cumin

¼ tsp. Cayenne pepper 1 tsp. Sea salt

½ tsp. Dry mustard

Barbecue Sauce

1 ½ cup mayonnaise

¼ cup apple cider vinegar 1 tbsp. English mustard

1 tsp. Black pepper 1 tsp. Salt

3 tsp. garlic , minced 2 tbsp. raw honey

2 tsp. Prepared horseradish

Combine all of the rub ingredients thoroughly.

Wash and dry the meat and take out any silver skin using a sharp knife.
Season the meat thoroughly with the rub mixture until the entire surface is coated.

Add the pork broth, apple cider vinegar and liquid smoke into the pressure cooker together with the meat and cook on high for 35 min.
Release the steam.

Combine all the sauce ingredients in a bowl and let it rest in the refrigerator for 3 hours. Preheat the oven to 450 degrees F.

Roast the meat for 6 minutes on each side or until crisp.

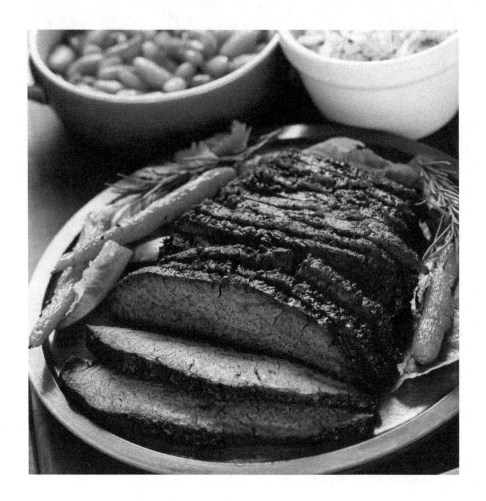

Spicy Maple Beef Brisket

Ingredients
3 lbs. beef brisket 1 cup pork broth
¼ cup apple cider vinegar 2 tsp. Liquid smoke
Rub Ingredients
1 tbsp. Maple Syrup
1 ½ tsp. Garlic powder 1 ½ tsp. Onion powder 1 ½ tsp. Black pepper
½ tsp. Hungarian Paprika 1 ½ tsp. Cumin
¼ tsp. Cayenne pepper 1 tsp. Sea salt
½ tsp. Dry mustard
Barbecue Sauce
1 ½ cup mayonnaise
¼ cup apple cider vinegar 1 tbsp. English mustard
1 tsp. Black pepper 1 tsp. Salt
3 tsp. garlic , minced 2 tbsp. raw honey
2 tsp. Prepared horseradish

Combine all of the rub ingredients thoroughly.
Wash and dry the meat and take out any silver skin using a sharp knife.
Season the meat thoroughly with the rub mixture until the entire
surface is coated.
Add the pork broth, apple cider vinegar and liquid smoke into the
pressure cooker together with the meat and cook on high for 35 min.
Release the steam.
Combine all the sauce ingredients in a bowl and let it rest in the
refrigerator for 3 hours. Preheat the oven to 450 degrees F.
Roast the meat for 6 minutes on each side or until crisp.

Chili Garlic Top Rump

Ingredients

3 lbs. Top rump 1 cup pork broth

¼ cup apple cider vinegar 2 tsp. Liquid smoke

Rub Ingredients

1 tbsp. Paprika

1 ½ tsp. Garlic powder 1 ½ tsp. Onion powder 1 ½ tsp. Black pepper

½ tsp. Chili powder 1 ½ tsp. Cumin

¼ tsp. Cayenne pepper 1 tsp. Sea salt

½ tsp. Dry mustard

Barbecue Sauce

1 ½ cup mayonnaise

¼ cup apple cider vinegar 1 tbsp. English mustard

1 tsp. Black pepper 1 tsp. Salt

3 tsp. garlic , minced 2 tbsp. raw honey

2 tsp. Prepared horseradish

Combine all of the rub ingredients thoroughly.

Wash and dry the meat and take out any silver skin using a sharp knife.
Season the meat thoroughly with the rub mixture until the entire
surface is coated.

Add the pork broth, apple cider vinegar and liquid smoke into the
pressure cooker together with the meat and cook on high for 35 min.
Release the steam.

Combine all the sauce ingredients in a bowl and let it rest in the
refrigerator for 3 hours. Preheat the oven to 450 degrees F.

Roast the meat for 6 minutes on each side or until crisp.

Italian Seared Flat Iron Steak

Ingredients
1 flat iron steak 2 tbsp. olive oil Sea Salt
1 Pinch of Italian Seasoning

Remove the meat from the refrigerator and pat dry and place on a rack for 15 min. Coat very thinly with oil.

The oil will hold the salt for the meat and it will also help conduct the heat to the meat. Sprinkle some ¼ tsp. of sea salt per side on the meat and rub it all over the meat.

Allow the meat to sit for 10 min. to allow the some of the juices to come out and give it a nice crust.

Heat some olive oil in your pan and sear the meat. Flip often until browned.

Let it rest for 10 min.

Sprinkle the rest of the ingredients.

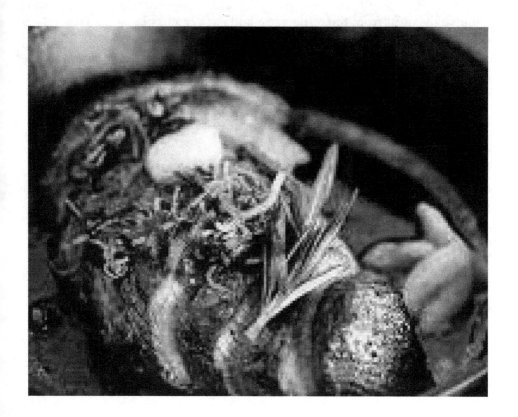

Seared Rib eye Steak with Rainbow Peppercorns

Ingredients
1 beef rib eye
2 tbsp. extra virgin olive oil Sea Salt
Freshly Ground Rainbow Peppercorns

Remove the meat from the refrigerator and pat dry and place on a rack for 15 min. Coat very thinly with oil.
The oil will hold the salt for the meat and it will also help conduct the heat to the meat. Sprinkle some ¼ tsp. of sea salt per side on the meat and rub it all over the meat.
Allow the meat to sit for 10 min. to allow the some of the juices to come out and give it a nice crust.
Heat some olive oil in your pan and sear the meat. Flip often until browned.
Let it rest for 10 min.
Sprinkle the rest of the ingredients.

Seared Rib eye Steak with Rainbow Peppercorns

Ingredients
1 beef rib eye
2 tbsp. extra virgin olive oil Sea Salt
Freshly Ground Rainbow Peppercorns

Remove the meat from the refrigerator and pat dry and place on a rack for 15 min. Coat very thinly with oil.
The oil will hold the salt for the meat and it will also help conduct the heat to the meat. Sprinkle some ¼ tsp. of sea salt per side on the meat and rub it all over the meat.
Allow the meat to sit for 10 min. to allow the some of the juices to come out and give it a nice crust.
Heat some olive oil in your pan and sear the meat. Flip often until browned.
Let it rest for 10 min.
Sprinkle the rest of the ingredients.

Simple Seared Porterhouse Steak

Ingredients
1 porterhouse steak
2 tbsp. extra virgin olive oil Sea Salt
Black Pepper

Remove the meat from the refrigerator and pat dry and place on a rack for 15 min. Coat very thinly with oil.
The oil will hold the salt for the meat and it will also help conduct the heat to the meat. Sprinkle some ¼ tsp. of sea salt per side on the meat and rub it all over the meat.
Allow the meat to sit for 10 min. to allow the some of the juices to come out and give it a nice crust.
Heat some olive oil in your pan and sear the meat. Flip often until browned.
Let it rest for 10 min.
Sprinkle the rest of the ingredients.

Italian Grilled T-Bone Steak

Ingredients

1 ½ lbs. T-bone steak Olive Oil

Seasoning Ingredients Sea Salt

1/2 tsp. Italian seasoning

1/2 tsp. ground black peppercorns

Preheat your grill or broiler to medium or medium high heat Cut the meat into slices fit for grilling.

Coat thinly with oil and sprinkle with the seasoning ingredients. Fold a strip of aluminum foil on the bones so that it doesn't burn. Cook the meat and flip every 20 seconds.

Take it out once the internal temperature of the meat reaches 138 to 145 degrees F. Let it rest for 5-10 min.

French Grilled Rib eye

Ingredients

1 ½ lbs. Rib eye Steak Olive Oil
Seasoning Ingredients Sea Salt
1/2 tsp. Herbs de Provence
1/2 tsp. ground rainbow peppercorns

Preheat your grill or broiler to medium or medium high heat Cut the meat into slices fit for grilling.

Coat thinly with oil and sprinkle with the seasoning ingredients. Fold a strip of aluminum foil on the bones so that it doesn't burn. Cook the meat and flip every 20 seconds.

Take it out once the internal temperature of the meat reaches 138 to 145 degrees F. Let it rest for 5-10 min.

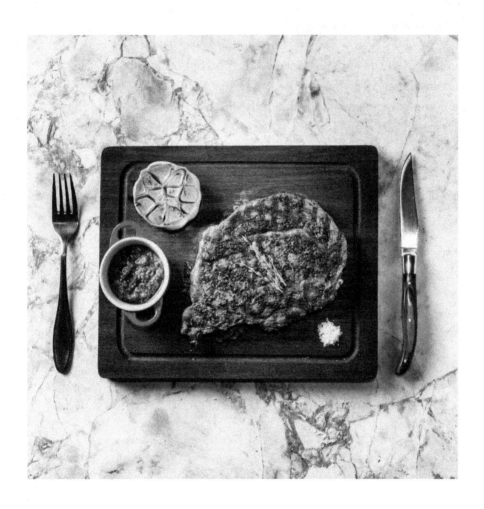

Chinese Poached Duck

Ingredients

1 distilled white vinegar Chicken Broth enough to cover 1 whole duck, quartered

Sea salt

4 ½ tsp. Sichuan peppercorns

Combine all of the ingredients in a large pot. Submerge the meat in liquid and heat to 180 degrees F.

You'll know the meat is done when the thermometer inserted to the thickest part of the thigh or breast reaches 155-165 degrees F.

Poached Turkey with Rainbow Peppercorns

Ingredients
1 distilled white vinegar Chicken Broth enough to cover 1 whole
turkey, quartered
Sea salt
4 ½ tsp. rainbow peppercorns

Combine all of the ingredients in a large pot. Submerge the meat in
liquid and heat to 180 degrees F.
You'll know the meat is done when the thermometer inserted to the
thickest part of the thigh or breast reaches 155-165 degrees F.

Spicy Poached Duck

Ingredients
1 distilled white vinegar Chicken Broth enough to cover 1 whole duck, quartered
Sea salt
2 ½ tsp. Chili Powder

Combine all of the ingredients in a large pot. Submerge the meat in liquid and heat to 180 degrees F.
You'll know the meat is done when the thermometer inserted to the thickest part of the thigh or breast reaches 155-165 degrees F.

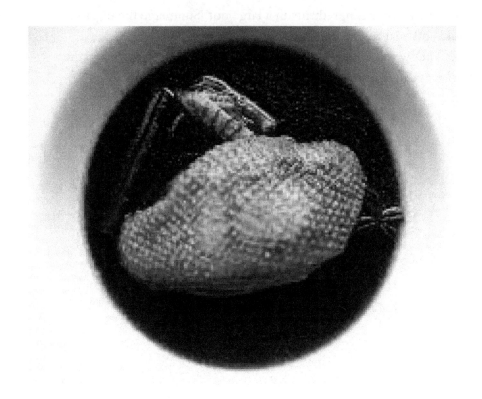

Asian Poached Turkey

Ingredients

1 distilled white vinegar Chicken Broth enough to cover 1 whole
turkey, quartered

Sea salt

4 ½ tsp. Sichuan peppercorns

Combine all of the ingredients in a large pot. Submerge the meat in
liquid and heat to 180 degrees F.

You'll know the meat is done when the thermometer inserted to the
thickest part of the thigh or breast reaches 155-165 degrees F.

Cold Rib eye

Ingredients

1 tbsp. finely chopped thyme leaves 2 tsp. Sage

3 tbsp. Olive Oil

2 ½-3 lbs. rib eye roast 1 tbsp. sea salt, to taste

Combine the sage and olive oil.

Rub it all over the beef and refrigerate overnight. Cook

Preheat the oven to 375 degrees F.

Rub the beef with salt and black pepper with your hands 20 min.

before roasting. Roast the beef for 15 min.

Turn the heat down to 325 degrees F and roast for 45 min. or until the

internal temperature shows 118 degrees F.

Let it rest for 45 min.

Wrap in plastic and put in the fridge.

Cut the beef into ½ inch thick slices and serve. Cook's Note:

This dish can last up to several days in your refrigerator and you can

use them for roast beef sandwiches.

When it comes to cooking thick cuts of meat like this, the meat

thermometer is your best friend.

When dealing with thick cuts of meat, make sure to season the surface

liberally with sea salt and black pepper.

Use coarse sea salt and black pepper on this one. It makes a huge

difference.

Minimalist Asparagus

Ingredients
1/4 cup water
1 lb. fresh asparagus, 1 inch cut off the bottom 1/2 tsp. sea salt

Spray some water onto paper towels or parchment paper and lay the asparagus on top. Sprinkle with salt and roll up the towels.
Lay the bundle seam side down in a microwave,
Cook
Microwave on high for 3-4 min. until crisp but tender.

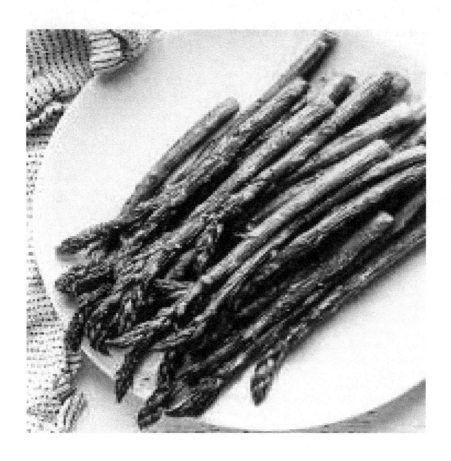

Baked Spinach Parsnips and Carrots

Ingredients
1/4 lb. fresh spinach, preferable blanched 1/4 lb. parsnips, cubed

1/4 lb. carrots, cubed

1/4 lb. turnips, cubed

3 tbsp. extra virgin olive oil 1 medium lemon, zested 1/2 tsp. sea salt

Preheat the oven to 500 degrees F.

Place all of the ingredients except the zest and salt in an aluminum foil.

Drizzle with oil and combine well.

Lay the vegetables in a single layer. Fold up the edges.

Cook

Bake for 5 min.

Toss the vegetables and bake again for 5 min. Sprinkle with zest and salt.

Baked Turnips Squash and Beets

Ingredients

1/4 lb. turnips, cubed

1/4 lb. summer squash, cubed 1/4 lb. beets, cubed

1/4 lb. parsnips, cubed 3 tbsp. olive oil

1 medium lime, zested

1/2 tsp. sea salt

Preheat the oven to 500 degrees F.

Place all of the ingredients except the zest and salt in an aluminum foil.

Drizzle with oil and combine well.

Lay the vegetables in a single layer. Fold up the edges.

Cook

Bake for 5 min.

Toss the vegetables and bake again for 5 min. Sprinkle with zest and salt.

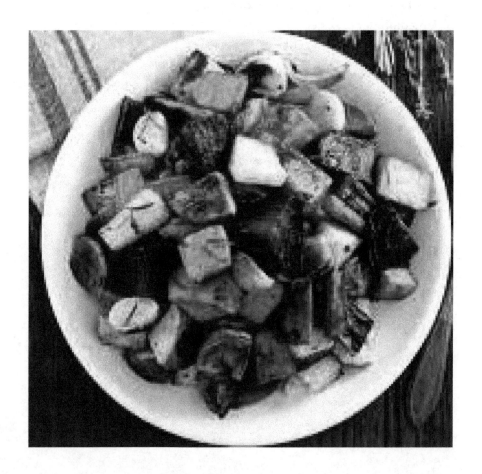

Smoky Poached Squash and Kohlrabi

Ingredients

1/2 lb. butternut squash, cubed 1/2 lb. kohlrabi

1/2 lb. red onion

1/3 cup low sodium vegetable broth Pinch kosher salt

2 tbsp. extra virgin olive oil 1/2 tsp. chili powder

1/2 tsp. smoked paprika

Place the vegetables on the bottom of a pan and add the water or broth and salt. Cover with lid and cook over high heat for 3 min.

Decrease the heat to low and cook for 3 min.

Remove from the heat and add the rest of the ingredients.

Spanish Poached Carrots and Parsnips

Ingredients

1/2 lb. carrots, cubed 1/2 lb. parsnips, cubed 1/2 lb. turnips, cubed
1/3 cup low sodium vegetable broth

Pinch sea salt

2 tbsp. extra virgin olive oil 1/2 tsp. Spanish paprika 1/2 tsp. annatto seeds

Place the vegetables on the bottom of a pan and add the water or broth and salt. Cover with lid and cook over high heat for 3 min.

Decrease the heat to low and cook for 3 min.

Remove from the heat and add the rest of the ingredients.

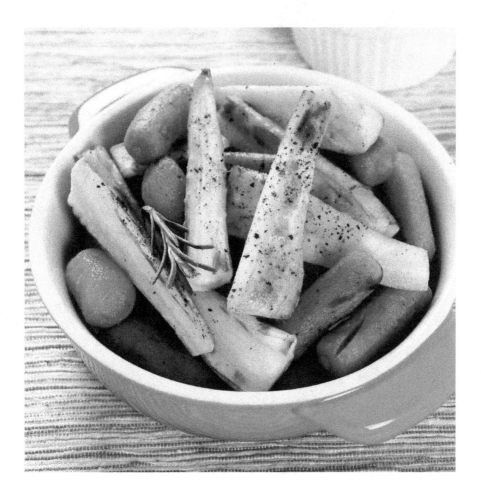

ALEX HENRY

CPSIA information can be obtained
at www.ICGtesting.com
Printed in the USA
BVHW090336040521
606332BV00006B/1015